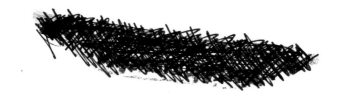

'VER' TY C   5T LONDO'

Royal Netherlands Academy of Arts and Sciences
P.O. Box 19121, 1000 GC Amsterdam, the Netherlands

Proceedings of the symposium,
Amsterdam, 9 – 11 April 1992

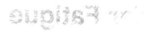

ISBN 0-444-85763-X

Koninklijke Nederlandse Akademie van Wetenschappen
Verhandelingen, Afd. Natuurkunde, Tweede Reeks, deel 91

Neuromuscular Fatigue

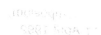

Edited by A.J. Sargeant and D. Kernell

North-Holland, Amsterdam/Oxford/New York/Tokyo, 1993

Contents

Section III *Long Term Processes: Usage Related Plasticity; Ageing; Damage*

Section IV *Muscle Performance: Mechanical Demand and Metabolic Supply*

Section V   *Neuronal Mechanisms and Processes*

Discussions

Foreword

Neuromuscular fatigue is a phenomenon of great importance in everyday life as well as being of great theoretical and clinical significance. Eleven years ago there was a seminal symposium on muscle fatigue held in London. The published proceedings (*Ciba Foundation Symposium 82 - "Human muscle fatigue: physiological mechanisms", Pitman, London, 1981*) served as an important 'state of the art' reference. In the intervening period there have been many developments with respect to our understanding of fatigue of the motor output, including processes located in the skeletal muscle fibres themselves as well as problems related to various aspects of (moto)neuronal muscle control. However, there are still uncertainties and important questions remain unanswered. We thought the time seemed ripe to attempt a renewed synthesis by bringing together international experts from a range of complementary research areas. In this way, we hoped, attention could be focussed on identifying the key questions that remain to be answered as well as providing an overview of already acquired answers and conclusions. We were fortunate to receive the opportunity to arrange an appropriate meeting as one of the series of "Academy Colloquia" of the *Royal Netherlands Academy of Arts and Sciences* (Koninklijke Nederlandse Akademie van Wetenschappen, KNAW).

We were happy to discover that our plans for a meeting on neuromuscular fatigue apparently were welcomed by our international colleagues; a high proportion of those invited also agreed to come. The symposium took place in Amsterdam during 9-11 April 1992. In accordance with the traditions for Academy Colloquia, the number of participants was limited to about 50; the program consisted of talks as well as poster presentations and much discussion (about 50% of the scheduled time). It should be stressed that, although there was time for only a rather limited number of oral presentations, the contributions of *all* participants were essential for the total impact and success of the meeting. The proceedings of the symposium are summarized in the present book which, we hope, will serve as a useful collective source of information concerning the multifaceted problems of neuromuscular fatigue.

We are very grateful to all those who helped, financially or otherwise, to make this symposium possible. Most of the costs and many of the organizational tasks were taken care of by the KNAW; important administrative contributions were delivered through the office of Drs. R. des Bouvrie (KNAW). Ms. M.M.M. Kooy (KNAW) and Ms. E. Verboom (Department of Muscle and Exercise Physiology) were largely responsible for the administrative organization of the meeting. We are also indebted to Dr. Arnold de Haan for both scientific and organizational advice. Furthermore, we were grateful to receive supplementary financial support from the Netherlands Organization for Scientific Research (NWO). The publication procedures were speeded up thanks to the rapidity with which the participants delivered their professionally formatted camera-ready manuscripts.

In the book, we have tried to arrange the various chapters in a more or less logical order according to subject matter. It should be stressed, however, that a perfect ordering of this kind would be impossible because, as might be expected, many of the contributions dealt with several different aspects of the complex subject matter of this symposium.

A.J.Sargeant   D.Kernell

List of participants

R. Bakels
University of Amsterdam
Dept. of Neurophysiology
Meibergdreef 15
1105 AZ Amsterdam
THE NETHERLANDS

P.R. Bär
University Hospital Utrecht
Research Laboratory Neurology
Heidelberglaan 100
3584 CX Utrecht
THE NETHERLANDS

A. Beelen
Vrije University & University of Amsterdam
Dept. of Muscle and Exercise Physiology
Meibergdreef 15
1105 AZ Amsterdam
THE NETHERLANDS

B. Bigland-Ritchie
Quinnipiac College and J.B. Pierce
Laboratory
290 Congress Avenue
New Haven
Connecticut 06519
U.S.A

R.A. Binkhorst
University of Nijmegen
Dept. of Physiology
Postbus 9101
6500 HB Nijmegen
THE NETHERLANDS

M.L. Blei
University of Washington
Department of Rehabilitation Medicine
Seattle
WA 98195
U.S.A.

A. De Haan
Vrije University & University of Amsterdam
Dept. of Muscle and Exercise Physiology
Meibergdreef 15
1105 AZ Amsterdam
THE NETHERLANDS

C.J. De Luca
Boston University
NeuroMuscular Research Center and
Dept. of Biomedical Engineering
44 Cummington Street
Boston, Massachusetts 02215
U.S.A.

C.J. De Ruiter
Vrije University & University of
Amsterdam
Dept. of Muscle and Exercise Physiology
Meibergdreef 15
1105 AZ Amsterdam
THE NETHERLANDS

H. Degens
University of Nijmegen
Dept. of Physiology
Postbus 9101
6500 HB Nijmegen
THE NETHERLANDS

J. Duchateau
Université Libre de Bruxelles
Laboratory of Biology
28 Avenue P. Héger
C.P. 168
1050 Brussels
BELGIUM

O. Eerbeek
University of Amsterdam
Department of Neurophysiology
Meibergdreef 15
1105 AZ Amsterdam
THE NETHERLANDS

R.M. Enoka
University of Arizona
Department of Exercise and Sports Sciences
Gittings Building
Tucson
AZ 85721
U.S.A.

J.A. Faulkner
The University of Michigan
Institute of Gerontology
Room 972-974, 300 N. Ingalls
Ann Arbor
Michigan 48109-0622
U.S.A

H.M. Franken
University of Twente
Dept. of Electrical Engineering
Postbus 217
7500 AE Enschede
THE NETHERLANDS

A.J. Fuglevand
University of Arizona
Department of Exercise and Sports
Sciences
Gittings Building
Tucson
AZ 85721
U.S.A.

S.C. Gandevia
The University of New South Wales
Department of Clinical Neurophysiology
Institute of Neurological Sciences
The Prince Henry Hospital and
Prince of Wales Research Institute
P.O. Box 233
Matraville, NSW 2036
AUSTRALIA

P.F. Gardiner
Université de Montréal
Département d'éducation physique
Case postale 6128
Succursale "A"
Montréal, Québec
CANADA   H3C 3J7

H. Gibson
University of Liverpool
Department of Medicine
Magnetic Resonance Research Center
and Muscle Research Center
P.O. Box 147, Liverpool L69 3BX
U.K.

T. Gordon
University of Alberta
Dept of Pharmacology and Division of
Neuroscience, Faculty of Medicine
525 Heritage Medical Research Center
Edmonton
CANADA   T6G 2H2

P.L. Greenhaff
University of Nottingham
Dept. of Physiology and Pharmacology
Queens Medical Centre
Nottingham NG7 2UH
U.K.

E. Hensbergen
University of Amsterdam
Department of Neurophysiology
Meibergdreef 15
1105 AZ Amsterdam
THE NETHERLANDS

D.A. Jones
University College London
Department of Physiology
Gower Street
London WC1E 6BT
U.K.

H.A. Keizer
Rijkuniversiteit Limburg
Department of Movement Sciences
P.O. Box 616
6200 MD Maastricht
THE NETHERLANDS

H.G.C. Kemper
Vrije University
Department of Health Sciences
Meibergdreef 15
1105 AZ Amsterdam
THE NETHERLANDS

D. Kernell
University of Amsterdam
Department of Neurophysiology
Meibergdreef 15
1105 AZ Amsterdam
THE NETHERLANDS

P.V. Komi
University of Jyväskyla
Dept. of Biology of Physical Activity
Rautpohjankatu 15
SF-40700 Jyvaskyla
FINLAND

H. Kuipers
Rijksuniversiteit Limburg
Department of Movement Sciences
P.O. Box 616
6200 MD Maastricht
THE NETHERLANDS

C.G. Kukulka
University of Rochester
Dept. of Physical Therapy
200 East River Road
Suite 1-102
Rochester NY 14623
U.S.A.

J. Lännergren
Karolinska Institutet
Department of Physiology II
S-104 01 Stockholm
SWEDEN

Y. Laouris
Cyprus Neuroscience & Technolog
Institute
Dept. of Neural Control
Lycourgou 10/401
Acropolis
Nicosia
CYPRUS

A. Lind
University of Amsterdam
Department of Neurophysiology
Meibergdreef 15
1105 AZ Amsterdam
THE NETHERLANDS

A.J. McComas
McMaster University
Health Sciences Centre
Department of Biomedical Sciences
1200 Main Street West
Hamilton, Ontario
CANADA L8N 3Z5

R.G. Miller
University of California
Dept. of Neurology
Tiburon
CA 94920
U.S.A.

M.V. Narici
Reparto di Fisiologia del Lavoro Muscolare
Instituto di Tecnologie Biomediche
Avanzate
Consiglio Nazionale delle Ricerche
Via Ampère, 56
20131 Milano
ITALY

B.W. Ongerboer de Visser
University of Amsterdam
Clinical Neurophysiology
Meibergdreef 9
1105 AZ Amsterdam
THE NETHERLANDS

L.C. Rome
University of Pennsylvania
Department of Biology
Philadelphia
PA 19104
U.S.A.

S. Salmons
University of Liverpool
Dept .of Human Anatomy and Cell Biology
British Heart Foundation Skeletal Muscle
Assist Research Group
P.O. Box 147, Liverpool L69 3BX
U.K.

B. Saltin
Karolinska Institutet
Department of Physiology III
Box 5626
S-114 86 Stockholm
SWEDEN

J.A.A. de Sant'Ana Pereira
Vrije University & University of
Amsterdam
Dept. of Muscle and Exercise Physiology
Meibergdreef 15
1105 AZ Amsterdam
THE NETHERLANDS

A.J. Sargeant
Vrije University & University of
Amsterdam
Dept. of Muscle and Exercise Physiology
Meibergdreef 15
1105 AZ Amsterdam
THE NETHERLANDS

N.C. Spurway
University of Glasgow
Institute of Physiology
G12 8QQ
U.K.

D.F. Stegeman
University of Nijmegen
Dept. of Neurology
Research Group on Neuromuscular
Disorders
Postbus 9101, 6500 HB Nijmegen
THE NETHERLANDS

D.G. Stuart
University of Arizona
College of Medicine
Department of Physiology
Health Sciences Center
Tucson, Arizona 85724
U.S.A

W.J. van der Laarse
Vrije University
Physiology Laboratory
Van der Boechorststraat 7
1081 BT Amsterdam
THE NETHERLANDS

P. Veltink
University of Twente
Dept. of Electrical Engineering
Postbus 217
7500 AE Enschede
THE NETHERLANDS

N.K. Vøllestad
Dept. of Physiology
National Institute of Occupational Health
P.O. Box 8149
N-0033 Oslo 1
NORWAY

W.A. Weijs
University of Amsterdam
Dept. of Functional Anatomy / ACTA
Meibergdreef 15
1105 AZ Amsterdam
THE NETHERLANDS

H.G. Westra
Vrije University
Dept. of Muscle and Exercise Physiology
Meibergdreef 15
1105 AZ Amsterdam
THE NETHERLANDS

C.A.T. Zijdewind
University of Amsterdam
Department of Neurophysiology
Meibergdreef 15
1105 AZ Amsterdam
THE NETHERLANDS

J.A. Zoladz
Academy of Physical Education
Dept. of Physiology & Biochemistry
Al. Jana Pawla II 62a
31-571 Cracow
POLAND

B. Zwaagstra
University of Amsterdam
Dept. of Neurophysiology
Meibergdreef 15
1105 AZ Amsterdam
THE NETHERLANDS

Section I

Cellular Processes of Muscle

Mechanisms of fatigue as studied in single muscle fibres

J. Lännergren, H. Westerblad & D.G. Allen

Department of Physiology II, Karolinska Institutet, 104 01 Stockholm, Sweden and Department of Physiology, University of Sydney, New South Wales, 2006, Australia.

Abstract Data from experiments on single, intact muscle fibres from Xenopus and mouse, aimed at elucidating cellular mechanisms of fatigue are summarized. During prolonged tetani there is evidence that conduction of action potentials down the t-tubuli may fail, leading to reduced Ca^{2+} release in the central part of the fibre. During repeated short tetani there is a uniform decline of Ca^{2+} across the fibre; in addition there is a reduction of force generating capacity of the crossbridges and diminished myofibrillar Ca^{2+} sensitivity. The possible relation of these alterations to changes in metabolite concentrations is discussed.

Muscle fatigue, here defined as a decline in force output during a period of activity, can be - and has been - studied in a number of different systems, from human athletes to minute myofibrillar preparations such as segments of 'skinned' muscle fibres. We have employed single, intact fibres for fatigue studies for the last 5-6 years. The advantage of this type of preparation is that adequate oxygenation is not a problem, the extracellular milieu can be controlled and changed rapidly if desired, and the action of drugs can be evaluated with high time resolution. Also, fibres of different types can be studied separately. It should be realized, however, that what we use is a *simplified model* of muscle fatigue and that in a whole muscle changes in the extracellular milieu are likely to contribute to fatigue development.

In the initial studies we used *amphibian* muscles because at that time this was the only kind which was amenable to single fibre dissection. We have used Xenopus muscle, because in this species fibres are relatively large and clearly differentiated into different types which can be identified and selected during the dissection. We chose to work on fibres from toe muscles (lumbricals) because these are short (1.5-1.8 mm) which facilitates electrical recordings. Lumbrical muscles contain fibres of amphibian types 1, 2, and 3, roughly corresponding to mammalian types IIb, IIa, and I, respectively. With time we developed a technique for dissecting single fibres from *mammalian* muscle as well (from mouse foot muscles) and results from experiments with such preparations will also be discussed.

Possible factors in fatigue

Signals for motor activity from the motor cortex are conveyed down the spinal cord to eventually activate motor neurons. Action potentials then travel out along motor nerve fibres, transmit across the neuromuscular junction and set up action potentials in the muscle fibres. Concomitant with the propagation along the surface membrane the action potential invades the t-tubules and triggers release of Ca^{2+} from adjacent regions of the sarcoplasmic reticulum (SR). This causes $[Ca^{2+}]_i$ to rise from a resting value of about 50 nM to 1-5 µM, which results in a conformational change in the troponin-tropomyosin complex occurs which then allows interaction of the mobile parts of myosin molecules (crossbridges) with actin, leading to force generation. Relaxation occurs when Ca^{2+} is pumped back from the myoplasm into the SR by an ATP-dependent Ca^{2+} pump in the wall of the SR.

It has been debated to what an extent the outflow of motor impulses from the CNS is reduced during fatiguing exercise. The concensus would appear to be that although such reductions can and do occur, the major site of fatigue is the muscle itself (Bigland-Ritchie & Woods 1984). In the experiments we are concerned with here, the fibres are activated directly with transverse field stimulation, which means that neither neuromuscular transmission nor surface propagation of action potentials will be a limiting factor.

1. Changes in action potential configuration

We found, as have others, that there are marked changes in the shape of the action potential especially with continuous, high frequency stimulation: the upstroke is less steep, the amplitude is reduced and repolarization is slowed down. However, an action potential of this altered configuration is still capable of eliciting a full-size, or even augmented, twitch (Lännergren & Westerblad 1986) from which it appears that this change, *per se*, is not a cause of fatigue.

2. Failure of t-tubule propagation

It has often been suggested that propagation of action potentials down the t-tubules is a weak link in activation (e.g. Jones 1981). Some of our experiments on Xenopus fibres give support for this idea (Lännergren & Westerblad 1986). With continuous high frequency stimulation (70 Hz) force stays up for about 5 s and then declines rapidly. Three lines of evidence point towards t-tubule failure as a cause for the decline in this case: i) the early negative after-potential (EAP) becomes less evident. The EAP is usually taken as a sign of electrical activity in the t-tubules; ii) force recovery is very rapid, either at the end of stimulation, or also *during* stimulation if the stimulus frequency is suddenly reduced. The rapid recovery time is compatible with restitution of the ionic milieu in the t-tubules; iii) intracellular Ca^{2+} release, as monitored with fura-2 and imaging microscopy, changes from being homogeneous in the beginning, when the force is high, to showing a clear radial gradient with less Ca^{2+} in the core of the fibre when tension goes down (Westerblad et al. 1990).

It is worth noting that in our experiments failure of inward spread of action potentials can occur at a normal extracellular K^+ concentration. In a whole working muscle blood flow is occluded even at moderate forces and K^+ will accumulate in the extracellular space, reaching levels of 9-12 mM in mammalian muscle (Juel 1986; Medbø & Sejersted 1990). The increase in $[K^+]_o$ will accentuate K^+ accumulation in the t-tubule lumen due to repeated action potentials. It is thus possible that even at moderate impulse frequencies t-tubule failure may develop in whole muscle and contribute to fatigue development.

3. Decreased Ca^{2+} release

Before discussing the possible contribution of failing Ca^{2+} release to fatigue it may be appropriate to briefly summarise current ideas about EC-coupling (t-tubule-SR transmission). The t-tubules and SR membranes are separated by a narrow space (width 10-15 nm) bridged by structures known as 'foot proteins'. The t-tubule membrane contains a modified Ca^{2+} channel (the dihydropyridine receptor) which acts as a voltage sensor. Depolarization of the membrane changes the conformation of the dihydropyridine receptor and this change affects a large protein complex which is both the foot protein and a Ca^{2+} channel in the SR membrane. The final result of t-tubule depolarization is opening of SR Ca^{2+} channels which allows Ca^{2+} to diffuse from the very high concentration in the SR to the much lower concentration in the myoplasm, removal of the steric block by the troponin-tropomyosin complex and start of the crossbridge cycle.

Experiments performed nearly 30 years ago by Eberstein and Sandow (1963) suggested failing EC-coupling to be an important fatigue mechanism. They found that caffeine could restore twitch force in single frog fibres which had been fatigued by a long period of twitching. Caffeine acts directly on SR Ca^{2+} channels and facilitates Ca^{2+} release (Rousseau et al. 1988). We repeated this type of experiment both on Xenopus and mouse fibres, fatigued by repeated tetanic stimulation and found in both cases that caffeine caused a dramatic force restoration (Westerblad & Lännergren 1986; Lännergren & Westerblad 1991). The result showed that in fatigue, the contractile machinery is still capable of substantial force production if sufficient Ca^{2+} release can be produced and suggested that failing Ca^{2+} release is an important mechanism of fatigue. Direct evidence for this view came from later experiments in which $[Ca^{2+}]_i$ was measured with aequorin (Allen et al. 1989) or with fura-2 in Xenopus fibres (Lee et al. 1991), later also in mouse fibres (Westerblad & Allen 1991). The change in amplitude of the Ca^{2+} transient during fatiguing, intermittent tetanic stimulation shows essentially the same pattern in Xenopus and mouse fibres. During the initial, fairly rapid period of tension decline to about 80% of the original the transient *increases,* it then slowly decreases while tension is relatively well maintained and then finally decreases markedly in parallel with a final, rapid tension decline (reviewed in Westerblad et al. 1991; see also Fig. 1). The importance of the reduction in Ca^{2+} release for the fall in tension is further substantiated by a concomitant increase in force and $[Ca^{2+}]_i$ when caffeine is applied (Westerblad & Allen 1991).

An important observation in studies of Ca^{2+} release in *Xenopus* fibres (Westerblad et al. 1990) was that with intermittent tetanic stimulation there was a *uniform* decline in $[Ca^{2+}]_i$ within fibres when force started to fall markedly, which indicates that t-tubule transmission does *not* fail in this fatigue model.

4. Reduced Ca^{2+} sensitivity of the contractile proteins

There are three principal mechanisms for reduced tension output in fatigue: i) reduced Ca^{2+} release; ii) reduced Ca^{2+} sensitivity of the contractile machinery; iii) reduced maximum force production by crossbridges. The first mechanism has just been discussed. As for the second possibility, experiments on skinned fibres have shown that metabolic changes which are likely to occur in fatigue, such as an increase in H^+ and P_i concentration, displace the curve relating force to $[Ca^{2+}]$ to the right, i.e. decrease the myofibrillar Ca^{2+} sensitivity (Godt & Nosek 1989). Recent experiments on mouse fibres by Westerblad and Allen (1991) show that at the end of a fatigue run, when force is down to about 35% of the original, the force-pCa curve is shifted by about 0.3 pCa units. Also in intact Xenopus fibres evidence for a diminished Ca^{2+} sensitivity was found (Lee et al. 1991).

5. Decreased force production by crossbridges

Several studies on 'skinned' fibre preparations have shown that the maximum force generation is depressed by metabolic changes which are likely to occur in fatigue. Thus, Cooke et al. (1988) and Godt & Nosek (1989) have demonstrated that a fall in pH from 7.0 to 6.5 together with an increase in P_i to 15 mM depresses maximum force by about 50%. Further, intracellular acidification of rested intact fibres by exposure to high CO_2 reduces maximum tension by 15-20% (e.g. Edman & Mattiazi, 1981).

Before discussing how the observed changes in tetanic force, Ca^{2+} release and Ca^{2+} sensitivity might relate to changes in metabolite concentrations a brief summary of such changes will be given, together with reference to some new data on metabolite concentrations in fatigued single Xenopus fibres.

Metabolite changes during fatigue

There is a wealth of data on metabolic changes during fatigue. The values obtained depend on various factors such as the preparation, type of fatiguing stimulation, aerobic/anaerobic conditions and so forth. Typical changes are a decrease in PCr from 35 to 2.4 mM, a decrease in ATP from 6 to 4.6 mM, an increase in P_i from 5 to 25 mM and a decrease in pH from 7.0 to 6.5 (reviewed by Vøllestad & Sejersted 1988; see also Godt & Nosek 1989; Westerblad et al. 1991). A recent study by Nagesser et al. (1992) is of particular relevance in the present context. They stimulated single Xenopus fibres (types 1 and 3) with intermittent tetani with a pattern similar to ours and measured, at various stages of fatigue, several metabolites of interest. Their findings are plotted in schematic form in Fig. 1. It can be seen that at 0.7-0-8 P_o, when tetanic force starts to fall rapidly, PCr is fully depleted, ATP starts to decrease and IMP starts to rise. At 0.3-0.4 P_o, the end-point of our fatigue runs, ATP is decreased by about 40%, P_i would have risen by about 30 mM, IMP has increased to ~2 mM and lactate to ~40 mM (type 1 fibres).

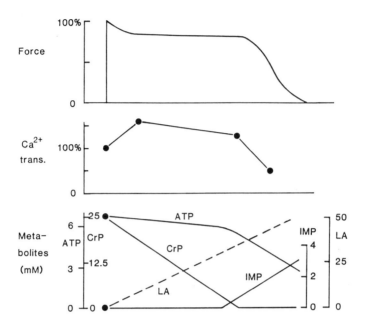

Fig. 1. Schematic representation of changes occurring in fatigue. Top panel: force production in repeated 70 Hz tetani; middle panel: amplitude of Ca^{2+} transients; bottom panel: metabolite concentrations. Metabolite values refer to Xenopus type 1 fibres. Data compiled from Westerblad & Allen (1991) and from Nagesser et al. (1992).

Possible relation between metabolite changes and force reducing mechanisms

It has long been recognized that there is a close correlation between metabolic capacity and the resistance to fatigue (eg. Kugelberg & Lindegren 1979). A very clear demonstration of this at the single fibre level was recently given by van der Laarse et al. (1991) where the time to fatigue (0.75 P_o) was related to the energy balance of Xenopus fibres of types 1-3, measured as SDH activity/myofibrillar ATPase activity, which gave a correlation coefficient of 0.93. The point of discussion is now how metabolite changes might have a bearing on the three cellular fatigue mechanisms referred to above and how they might develop with time.

i) Reduced force generation of cross-bridges. This change develops early as indicated by the finding that when force has fallen to about 0.8 P_o (after 10-20 tetani), caffeine application does not give any force enhancement. The most likely candidates for force depression, P_i and H^+, have already been discussed above. It should be pointed out here that isolated mouse fibres show little pH change in fatigue produced by repeated tetani (Westerblad & Allen 1992) so for these fibres P_i would be the dominant factor.

Mechanisms of fatigue as studied in single muscle fibres

ii) Reduced Ca²⁺ sensitivity. Force-pCa curves have mainly been measured towards the end of fatiguing stimulation, i.e. when force is down to 0.3-0.4 P_o, and compared with resting conditions so it is not possible to state in detail how sensitivity changes with time. Judging from skinned fibre results the metabolic changes which are most likely to be responsible are inceases in P_i and H^+, similar to the case of maximum force depression.

iii) Reduced Ca²⁺ release. In our experimental model there was evidence for failing t-tubule function during a prolonged tetanus at high frequency, but *not* with repeated tetanic stimulation. In principle, a homogeneous depression of Ca^{2+} release might be due to either a decreased Ca^{2+} content of the SR or inhibition of the release mechanism. The finding that caffeine can release substantial amounts of Ca^{2+} in fatigued fibres is difficult to reconcile with SR depletion. Further, electron probe microanalysis of the ionic content of the SR of fatigued fibres failed to show a decrease in Ca^{2+} concentration (Gonzalez-Serratos et al. 1978).

Considering the second possibility, i.e. failure of Ca^{2+} release, Fig. 1 suggests that the failure might be connected with metabolic changes. One suggestive point is that the marked fall in the amplitude of the Ca^{2+} transient coincides with the time when ATP starts to decline. ATP is known to be required for the opening of SR Ca^{2+} channels (Smith et al. 1985), but it appears that also ADP and AMP can fulfil this role, at least for channels incorporated into artificial membranes. However, it has recently been demonstrated that phosphorylation of the voltage-sensitive DHP-channels in the t-tubules increases their readiness to open in response to depolarization (Mundina-Weilenmann et al. 1991). It is conceivable that phosphorylation also of the SR Ca^{2+}-channels is important for their opening probability, thus giving the phosphorylation potential ($[ATP]/[ADP][P_i]$ ratio) in the vicinity of the channels a possible functional role.

A second feature of the metabolic changes depicted in Fig. 1 is that decreased Ca^{2+} release coincides with a rise in IMP concentration. The effect of IMP on channel opening appears not to have been investigated but it cannot be excluded that it has an inhibitory effect.

A consequence of the fall in ATP is that cytoplasmic $[Mg^{2+}]$ will rise since ATP forms a complex with Mg^{2+} with a higher binding constant than for other nucleotides. Westerblad & Allen (1992) have shown that free $[Mg^{2+}]_i$ does indeed rise during the final phase of a fatigue run. This is of particular interest since it has been demonstrated by Lamb and Stephenson (1991) that an increase of $[Mg^{2+}]$ from its normal resting value of 1 mM to 3 mM significantly inhibits Ca^{2+} release from semi-intact fibre preparations. A direct test of the Mg^{2+} inhibition hypothesis by injection of Mg^{2+} into intact mouse fibres showed that the inhibition was not large enough to explain the tension reduction in fatigue. However, the combination of increasecd Mg^{2+} and low ATP might be more effective in inhibiting Ca^{2+} release.

Yet another connection between a fall in ATP and reduced Ca^{2+} release might be provided by ATP-sensitive K^+ channels which exist in skeletal muscle (Spruce et al 1987). These channels are opened at low $[ATP]_i$, augmenting K^+ efflux (Castle & Haylett 1987) and changing the shape of the action potential (Sauviat et al 1991) which could lead to impaired activation of the Ca^{2+} release channels by the t-tubule voltage sensors.

Previous experiments on isolated Ca^{2+} channels in artificial membranes indicated that their opening probability is greatly reduced by low pH (Ma et al. 1988). However, using mechanically skinned fibres, where channels remain in a more natural environment, Lamb et al. (1992) have shown that acidosis in all likelihood has very little effect on Ca^{2+} release under physiological conditions. Thus, a fall in pH_i, as observed especially in amphibian type 1 fibres (but not in mouse fibres, see above) does not depress force via interference with Ca^{2+} release but more likely through an effect at the crossbridge level.

Relevance of single fibre studies

The results summarized here are all derived from experiments on isolated fibres. A question which naturally arises is how representative they are for fatigue in vivo. One factor which differs is that in the single fibre experiments the preparation is continuously superfused with fresh solution so that the extracellular environment remains constant. In whole muscles, on the other hand, blood flow is impeded already during moderate contractions, which means that substances such as lactic acid and K^+ ions will accumulate in the extracellular space. These changes in extracellular composition may aggravate some of the fatigue mechanisms described. For instance, changes in pH_i are likely to be more pronounced than we have observed and ionic changes in the t-tubule lumen may occur more readily, increasing the risk of failure of inward spread of action potentials. On the other hand, in single fibre experiments the extracellular milieu can be modified in a controlled way, allowing a systematic analysis of the contribution of extracellular changes to the development of muscle fatigue.

References

Allen DG, Lee JA & Westerblad H (1989). Intracellular calcium and tension in isolated single muscle fibres from Xenopus. *Journal of Physiology* **415**, 433-458.

Bigland-Ritchie B & Woods JJ (1984). Changes in muscle contractile properties and neural control during human muscular fatigue. *Muscle & Nerve* **7**, 691-699.

Castle NA & Haylett DG (1987). Effect of channel blockers on potassium efflux from metaboilically exhausted frog skeletal muscle. *Journal of Physiology* **383**, 31-43.

Cooke R, Franks K, Luciani GB & Pate E (1988). The inhibition of rabbit skeletal muscle contraction by hydrogen ion and phosphate. *Journal of Physiology* **345**, 77-97.

Eberstein A & Sandow A (1963). Fatigue mechanisms in muscle fibres. In: *The Effect of Use and Disuse on Neuromuscular Functions*. Elsevier. Amsterdam. pp 515-526

Edman KAP & Mattiazzi AR (1981). Effects of fatigue and altered pH on isometric force and velocity of shortening at zero load in frog muscle fibres. *Journal of Muscle Research and Cell Motility* **2**, 321-334.

Godt RE & Nosek TM (1989). Changes of intracellular milieu with fatigue or hypoxia depress contraction of striated rabbit skeletal and cardiac muscle. *Journal of Physiology* **412**, 155-180.

Gonzalez-Serratos H, Somlyo AV, McClellan G, Shuman H, Borrero LM & Somlyo AP (1978). Composition of vacuoles and sarcoplasmic reticulum in fatigued muscle: electron probe analysis. *Proceedings of the National Academy of Science (USA)* **75**, 1329-1333.

Juel C (1986). Potassium and sodium shifts during in vitro isometric contraction, and the time course of the ion-gradient recovery. *Pflügers Archiv* **406**, 458-463

Jones DA (1981). Muscle fatigue due to changes beyond the neuromuscular junction. In: Human Muscle Fatigue: Physiological Mechanisms (Ciba Foundation Symposium 82) Eds, Porter R and Whelan J. Pitman Medical. London. pp 178-196

Kugelberg E & Lindegren B (1979). Transmission and contractile fatigue of rat motor units in relation to succinate dehydrogenase activity of motor unit fibres. *Journal of Physiology* **288**, 285-300.

Lamb GD & Stephenson DG (1991). Effect of Mg^{2+} on the control of Ca^{2+} release in skeletal muscle fibres of the toad. *Journal of Physiology* **434**, 507-528.

Lamb GD, Recupero E & Stephenson (1992). Effect of myoplasmic pH on excitation-contraction coupling in skeletal muscle fibres of the toad. *Journal of Physiology* **448**, 211-224.

Lännergren J & Westerblad H (1986). Force and membrane potential during and after fatiguing, continuous high frequency stimulation of single Xenopus muscle fibres. *Acta Physiologica Scandinavica* **128**, 359-368.

Lännergren J & Westerblad H (1991). Force decline due to fatigue and intracellular acidification in isolated fibres from mouse skeletal muscle. *Journal of Physiology* **434**, 307-322.

Lee JA, Westerblad H & Allen DG (1991). Changes in tetanic and resting $[Ca^{2+}]_i$ during fatigue and recovery of single muscle fibres from Xenopus laevis. *Journal of Physiology* **415**, 433-458.

Ma J, Fill M, Knudson M, Campbell KP & Coronado R (1988). Ryanodine receptor of skeletal muscle is a gap junction-type channel. *Science* **242**, 99-102.

Medbø JI & Sejersted OM (1990). Plasma potassium changes with high intensity exercise. *Journal of Physiology* **421**, 105-122.

Mundina-Weilenmann C, Ma J, Rios E & Hosey MM (1991). Dihydropyridine sensitive skeletal muscle channels in polarized bilayers. 2. Effects of phosphorylation by a cAMP-dependent protein kinase. *Biophysical Journal* **60**, 902-909.

Nagesser AS, van der Laarse WJ & Elzinga G (1992). Metabolic changes with fatigue in different types of single muscle fibres of Xenopus laevis. *Journal of Physiology* **448**, 511-523.

Rousseau E, LaDine J, Lin Q-Y & Meissner G (1988). Activation of the Ca^{2+} release channel of skeletal muscle sarcoplasmic reticulum by caffeine and related compounds. *Archives of Biochemistry and Biphysics* **267**, 75-86.

Sauviat M-P, Ecault E, Faivre J-F & Findlay I (1991). Activation of ATP-sensitive K channels by a K channel opener (SR 44866) and the effect upon electrical and mechanical activity of frog skeletal muscle. *Pflügers Archiv* **418**, 261-265.

Smith JS, Coronado R & Meissner G (1985). Sarcoplasmic reticulum contains adenine nucleotide-activated calcium channels. *Nature* **316**, 446-449.

Spruce AE, Standen NB & Stanfield PR (1985). Voltage-dependent ATP-sensitive potassium channels of skeletal muscle membrane. *Nature* **316**, 736-738.

van der Laarse WJ, Lännergren J & Diegenbach PC (1991). Resistance to fatigue of single muscle fibres from Xenopus related to succinate dehydrogenase and myofibrillar ATPase activities. *Experimental Physiology* **76**, 589-596.

Vøllestad NK & Sejersted OM (1988). Biochemical correlates of fatigue. *European Journal of Applied Physiology* **57**, 336-347.

Westerblad H & Lännergren J (1987). Tension restoration with caffeine in fatigued, single Xenopus muscle fibres of various types. *Acta Physiologica Scandinavica* **130**, 357-358.

Westerblad H, Lee JA, Lamb AG, Bolsover SR & Allen DG (1990). Spatial gradients of intracellular calcium in sketal muscle during fatigue. *Pflügers Archiv* **415**, 734-740.

Westerblad H & Allen DG (1991). Changes of myoplasmic calcium concentration during fatigue in single mouse muscle fibers. *Journal of General Physiology* **98**, 615-635.

Westerblad H, Lee JA, Lännergren J & Allen DG (1991). Cellular mechanisms of fatigue in skeletal muscle. *American Journal of Physiology* **261**, C195-C209.

Westerblad H & Allen DG (1992) Changes of intracellular pH due to repetitive stimulation of single fibres from mouse skeletal muscle. *Journal of Physiology* **449**, 49-71.

Westerblad H & Allen DG (1992). Myoplasmic free Mg^{2+} concentration during repetitive stimulation of single muscle fibres from mouse skeletal muscle. *Journal of Physiology* (in press).

Determination of the rate of ATP hydrolysis during the development of fatigue in single muscle fibres

W.J. van der Laarse and A.S. Nagesser

Laboratorium voor Fysiologie, Vrije Universiteit, Van der Boechorststraat 7, 1081 BT Amsterdam, The Netherlands

Experiments on skinned muscle fibres indicate that loss of mechanical performance of fatigued muscle is due to increased inorganic phosphate concentration and acidification (Chase & Kushmerick, 1988; Cooke et al., 1988; Godt & Nosek, 1989), whereas experiments on intact fibres indicate that reduced calcium efflux from the sarcoplasmic reticulum is the most important force-reducing mechanism (Allen et al., 1989). To investigate the relative importance of the various mechanisms responsible for reduced mechanical performance, which may all relate to energetic properties of muscle fibres, we have determined metabolite contents (phosphocreatine, creatine, ATP, IMP), lactate production, and oxygen uptake of single, intact muscle fibres. These data are used here to determine the relationship between force production and the rate of ATP hydrolysis during the development of fatigue induced by intermittent tetanic stimulation.

Methods

Single, intact, fast-twitch, low oxidative (type 1) muscle fibres were dissected from the iliofibularis muscle of *Xenopus laevis* (Lännergren and Smith, 1966). They were stimulated intermittently at 40 Hz to produce one 250 ms tetanus every 5 s in oxygenated, phosphate buffered Ringer solution, pH 7.2, at 20 °C. Oxygen uptake of three fibres was determined as described by Elzinga and van der Laarse (1988). Nineteen fibres were freeze-clamped after different stimulation times (0, 1.5, 4, 5 and 10 min, n = 3 to 5) and used to determine metabolite contents as described by Nagesser et al. (1992). Lactate efflux was also determined. From these data the amount of energy-rich phosphate (~P) utilized was calculated using ~P/ATP = 2 (because ATP is converted to IMP), ~P/lactate = 1.5 and ~P/O_2 = 6.3.

Results and Discussion

Fig. 1 shows that the rate of ATP hydrolysis is not proportional to force production (contrary to results of Dawson et al., 1978): after a fairly proportional decrease during the first 5 min of intermittent stimulation (coinciding with full reduction of the phosphocreatine store and an increase of lactate content to 145 μmol.g^{-1} dry weight, results not shown), the rate of ATP hydrolysis decreases faster than force. The rate of ATP hydrolysis must fall because ATP regeneration in the sarcoplasm (from phosphocreatine and by glycolysis) is almost fully reduced and the rate of oxygen consumption cannot increase further: during this phase and beyond virtually all ATP is regenerated by oxidative phosphorylation. Mitochondrial capacity is too low to maintain the high rate of ATP hydrolysis. ATP is not depleted to compensate for the reduced rate of ATP production, but is converted slowly to IMP. When the low, steady rate of ATP hydrolysis is reached, force decreases rapidly. This major force reduction is probably due to decreased calcium efflux from the sarcoplasmic reticulum (Allen et al., 1989).

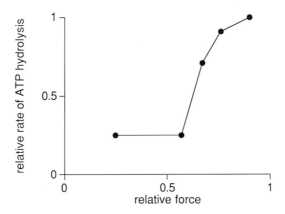

Figure 1. The rate of ATP hydrolysis during five time intervals of fatiguing intermittent stimulation (see Methods) plotted against the mean force production during the time intervals. The initial rate of ATP hydrolysis during contraction is 9 nmol.mm^{-3}.s^{-1}, corresponding to about 7 mM per 250 ms tetanus in the overlap zone of actin and myosin filaments.

The results are compatible with the idea that the rate of ATP hydrolysis is inhibited first by inorganic phosphate and protons (Cooke et al., 1988) and subsequently by ADP, which is expected to rise during contraction when ATP regeneration in the sarcoplasm is reduced.

References

Allen DG, Lee JA & Westerblad H (1989). Intracellular calcium and tension during fatigue in isolated single muscle fibres from *Xenopus laevis*. *Journal of Physiology* **415**, 433-458.

Chase PB & Kushmerick MJ (1988). Effects of pH on contraction of rabbit fast and slow skeletal muscle fibers. *Biophysical Journal* **53**, 935-946.

Cooke R, Franks K, Luciani GB & Pate E (1988). The inhibition of rabbit skeletal muscle contraction by hydrogen ions and phosphate. *Journal of Physiology* **395**, 77-97.

Dawson MJ, Gadian DG & Wilkie DR (1978). Muscular fatigue investigated by phosphorus nuclear magnetic resonance. *Nature* **274**, 861-866.

Elzinga G & van der Laarse WJ (1988). Oxygen consumption of single muscle fibres of *Rana temporaria* and *Xenopus laevis* at 20°C. *Journal of Physiology* **399**, 405-418.

Godt RE & Nosek TM (1989). Changes of intercellular milieu with fatigue or hypoxia depress contraction of skinned rabbit skeletal and cardiac muscle. *Journal of Physiology* **412**, 155-180.

Lännergren J & Smith R (1966). Types of muscle fibres in toad skeletal muscle. *Acta Physiologica Scandinavica* **68**, 263-274.

Nagesser AS, van der Laarse WJ & Elzinga G (1992). Metabolic changes with fatigue in different types of single muscle fibres of *Xenopus laevis*. *Journal of Physiology* **448**, 511-523.

Normal range of ATPase and ATP synthesis rates of human skeletal muscle determined noninvasively by a QUantitative Energetic Stress Test

M.L. Blei[1], K.E. Conley[2], and M.J. Kushmerick[2,3]

Department of Rehabilitation Medicine[1], UCHSC, Denver, Colorado and Departments of Radiology[2], Physiology and Biophysics[3], University of Washington, Seattle, Washington, USA.

Human skeletal muscle is well known to be composed of a heterogeneous population of muscle fibers with respect to ATPase activity, aerobic capacity, and fatigue resistance. Further, significant heterogeneity between fiber-types has been demonstrated in the resting metabolic profile of other mammalian skeletal muscles. In addition, human voluntary contractions follow an orderly recruitment of motor units. The degree of spacial recruitment during steady-state voluntary contractions will be correlated to the extent of neuromuscular fatigue developing in the initially activated motor units. These issues complicate the in vivo study of human skeletal muscle energetics.

The evaluation of chemical energetics in skeletal muscle has been significantly advanced within the last decade largely because of applications of ^{31}P magnetic resonance spectroscopy (MRS) techniques (Arnold,Matthews, & Radda, 1984; Chance,Leigh,Clark,Maris,Kent,Nioka, et al., 1986). The QUantitative Energetic Stress Test (QUEST) recently developed for the evaluation of human skeletal muscle was designed to i) measure separately ATP utilization from ATP synthesis, ii) control cytosolic conditions with respect to pH, and iii) minimize the variabilities associated with normal physiologic motor unit recruitment and fatigue development upon the measure (Blei,Kushmerick,Esselman, & Odderson, 1991).

Methods

Percutaneous, supramaximal twitch stimulation (1 Hz) of the median and ulnar nerves was applied in combination with ischemia to the finger and wrist flexors in 8 normal subjects during 3 repeated measures. The experiments utilized a 2.0 Tesla General Electric CSI spectrometer with continuous ^{31}P Magnetic Resonance Spectroscopy (MRS) acquisition. The protocol and data acquizition have been previously described (Blei et al., 1991). The sequential spectrum were analized using a least squares comparison with a high signal-to-noise spectrum referenced to a quantified fully-relaxed spectrum.

Results

The duration of the ischemia (360 sec) preceding the ischemic stimulation was sufficient to deplete the muscle oxygen stores. During the 1 Hz stimulation train, the mean initial rate of phosphocreatine (PCr) breakdown was 0.40% baseline [PCr]/sec ($\pm 0.07\%$/sec SD). The mean relative standard deviation of 3 repeated measures for an individual was 9%. The mean initial rate of depletion during stimulation significantly differed among subjects (ANOVA, $P<0.0003$) with a range of 1.7 fold. Small changes in pH were recorded, yet the mean pH did not exceed the range of 7.07 to 6.95 during the experiments. After a brief time delay, the recovery process approximated a monoexponential time course; however, the maximum PCr/(PCr + Pi) significantly overshot ($93.7\% \pm 3.5\%$ SD) the pre-stimulation control level ($88.9\% \pm 2.3\%$ SD; $P<0.0001$, paired t-test, n=24). The recovery time constant averaged 59.8 sec (± 13.7 sec SD) for the eight subjects with a mean relative standard deviation of 3 repeated measurements for an individual of 9%. The mean recovery time constants significantly differed among the eight subjects (ANOVA, $P<0.0001$) with a range of 1.9 fold.

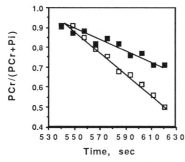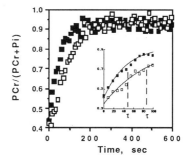

Figure 1. A) Range of initial rates of ATP utilization, and B) Range of recovery time constants in the eight normal subjects.

Discussion

The experimental protocol is able to achieve reproducible, independent, quantitative measures of high energy phosphate utilization and synthesis in human skeletal muscle. With respect to each energetic characteristic, it is capable of making statistical distinctions between individuals

The results demonstrate a predicted degree of intersubject variation. The human vastus lateralis has been previously shown to have a similar fiber-type distribution as the forearm flexors (Johnson,Polgar,Weightman, & Appleton, 1973). Utilizing biopsy data from the human vastus lateralis, the estimated range of energy utilization would vary 1.7 fold assuming simply a constant [PCr] among fiber-types and two fiber populations varying between 30-70% ST with a five fold difference in ATPase activity (Bárány, 1967; Chase & Kushmerick, 1988; Howald,Hoppeler,Claassen,Mathieu, & Straub, 1985; Johnson et al., 1973). Mitochondrial volume density in the vastus lateralis ranges from 4-7% or 1.75 fold. (Howald et al., 1985). These closely estimate the intersubject variability seen in our utilization data (1.7 fold) and recovery data (1.9 fold). In addition, the correlation between the calculated mean relative ATP utilization rates and synthesis time constants is: r = 0.45, p<.05, n=8; whereas, in Howald's data the correlation between fiber-types and mitochondrial volume density was: r = 0.42, n=10 (unpublished results). These results demonstrate the power of QUEST as a non-invasive biopsy of skeletal muscle composition and its potential in the serial monitoring of adaptation during specific training regimens and during pathological interventions.

References

Arnold DL, Matthews PM, & Radda GK (1984). Metabolic recovery after exercise and the assessment of mitochondrial function in vivo in human skeletal muscle by means of 31P NMR. *Magnetic Resonance in Medicine, 1*(3), 307-15.

Bárány M (1967). ATPase activity of myosin correlated with speed of muscle shortening. *Journal of General Physiology, 50*(6), 197-218.

Blei ML, Kushmerick MJ, Esselman P & Odderson I (1991). Pattern of Normal Human Muscle Energetics Utilizing a New Quantitative Exercise Stress Test (QUEST) Protocol. Tenth Annual Society of Magnetic Resonance in Medicine Meeting, 110a, San Fransisco, CA.

Chance B, Leigh JJ, Clark BJ, Maris J, Kent J, Nioka S & Smith D (1986). Multiple controls of oxidative metabolism in living tissues as studied by phosphorus magnetic resonance. *Proceedings of the National Academy of Science U S A, 83*(24), 9458-62.

Chase BP & Kushmerick MJ (1988). Effects of pH on Contraction of Rabbit Fast and Slow Skeletal Muscle Fibers. *Biophysical Journal, 53*, 935-946.

Howald H, Hoppeler H, Claassen H, Mathieu O & Straub R (1985). Influences of endurance training on the ultrastructural composition of the different muscle fiber types in humans. *Pflugers Archives European Journal of Physiology, 403*(4), 369-76.

Johnson MA, Polgar J, Weightman D & Appleton D (1973). Data on the distribution of fibre types in thirty-six human muscles. An autopsy study. *Journal of the Neurological Sciences, 18*(1), 111-29.

Reduced tetanic calcium in fatigue of whole skeletal muscle

A.J.Baker, M.C.Longuemare, R.Brandes, M.W.Weiner & R.G Miller[*]

Depts. Medicine, Radiology, and [*]Neurology, Univ. California, San Francisco. VA Medical Center. 4150 Clement Street, San Francisco, Ca 94121. & [*]California Pacific Medical Center.

One mechanism of fatigue may be that the rise of intracellular calcium (Ca^{2+}_i) during contraction of fatigued muscle is not sufficient to fully activate the contractile proteins (1-3). Studies of calcium in single skeletal muscle fibers using Ca^{2+}-sensitive indicators suggested fatigue was associated with reduced tetanic $[Ca^{2+}]_i$ (1-3). The present study aimed to determine in a whole muscle if there is a relationship between altered contractility during fatigue and changes of cytosolic free calcium. The approach was to measure the tetanic force of whole bullfrog semitendinosus muscles while monitoring calcium with the Ca^{2+}-sensitive fluorescent indicator Indo-1. These whole muscle experiments extend previous single cell studies of fatigue and $[Ca^{2+}]_i$ (1-3) in several directions. First, while fatigue has been extensively studied in whole muscle, no studies have monitored changes of $[Ca^{2+}]_i$ and force during fatigue of whole muscle. Second, calcium measurements with Indo-1 have important advantages in minimizing artifacts due to motion of the preparation, leakage or bleaching of indicator during the experiment, or differences in indicator concentration between experiments. Indo-1 has not yet been exploited to monitor calcium in contracting whole skeletal muscle. Finally, with the high signal to noise fluorescence measurements obtainable from whole muscle, it was possible to quantitate the relaxation phase of the calcium signal. A slowing of force relaxation with fatigue is well known. However, quantitative relationships between changes in both force- and calcium relaxation with fatigue have not yet been defined.

Experimental methods

Bullfrog semitendinosus muscles were loaded with the calcium-sensitive indicator Indo-1 by arterial perfusion with an oxygenated loading solution consisting of Ringer, Indo-1-AM (5 µm), calf serum (5%), probenecid (1 mM), pluronic acid (2%) and dimethyl sulfoxide (1%), for 40 min at 4 ml/hr and 30°C. Indo-1-loaded muscles were set near the twitch-optimum length and supramaximally stimulated through parallel wire electrodes placed on either side of the muscle. Force and calcium (inferred from Indo-1 fluorescence) were measured during tetani (0.1 ms pulses at 100 Hz for 200 ms) at various levels of fatigue induced by repeated stimulation. Indo-1 fluorescence was recorded using a SLM 48000S spectrofluorometer. Indo-1-loaded muscles were illuminated at 350 nm through a fiber optic cable and the fluorescence intensity of the muscle was measured at 400 nm and 470 nm. Changes in calcium were inferred from changes in the ratio (R) of 400/470 nm intensities. During relaxation, time constants for the fall in force and R were calculated from a least squares fit to exponential expressions.

Results

Figure 1 shows that tetanic stimulation (indicated by the horizontal line) caused fluorescence to increase at 400 nm (I_{400}) and decrease at 470 nm (I_{470}). Changes of $[Ca^{2+}]_i$ were inferred from the ratio (R) of I_{400}/I_{470} (Fig. 1). Artifacts due to motion or changes of indicator content have similar relative effects at each wavelength and therefore cancel in the ratio. The rise of $[Ca^{2+}]_i$ started almost immediately after stimulation and preceded force development. During the tetanus, $[Ca^{2+}]_i$ rapidly reached a steady state and remained almost constant while force increased. The fall of $[Ca^{2+}]_i$ started soon after the end of stimulation and preceded the fall of force. Figure 2 shows the relationship between force and R during fatigue (means ± std error, n=7). Progressive decreases of R were accompanied by proportional decreases of force. Fatigue also resulted in a slowing of the rate at which both force and calcium relaxed at the end of the stimulation. Figure 3 shows that the time constants of relaxation of force and R both increased in parallel as force decreased with fatigue.

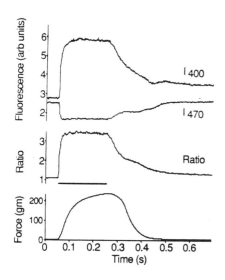

Fig. 1. Typical records of fluorescence at 400nm, 470nm, their ratio (reflecting Ca^{2+}) and force during a tetanus (horizontal bar).

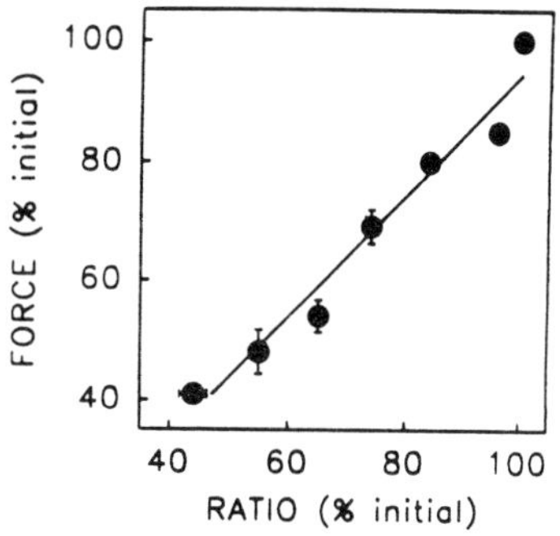

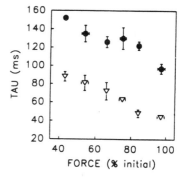

Fig. 2. Decreased force and R (reflecting Ca^{2+}) during fatigue (means ± std err n=7).

Fig. 3. (at right). Increases of relaxation time constants of force (▼) and R (•) with fatigue (means ± std err n=4).

Discussion

There were two major findings. First, fatiguing stimulation of whole skeletal muscle caused proportional decreases of force and R. This suggests that intracellular calcium was diminished with fatigue and therefore a component of the decrease in force may arise from a decrease in the tetanic level of calcium available to activate the contractile proteins. Second, fatiguing stimulation caused progressive slowing of relaxation of force and R. This suggests that relaxation of calcium was slowed with fatigue and therefore slowed force relaxation with fatigue may be mediated by slowed sequestration of calcium from the myoplasm. In conclusion, the findings of this study are consistent with measurements from single fibers and suggest that changes in calcium handling may play a significant role in the fatigue produced by intermittent tetanic stimulation.

References

1. Allen DG, JA Lee & H. Westerblad. Intracellular calcium and tension during fatigue in isolated single muscle fibers from xenopus laevis. *J. Physiol.* 415: 433-458, 1989.
2. Lee JA, H Westerblad & DG Allen. Changes in tetanic and resting $[Ca^{2+}]_i$ during fatigue and recovery of single muscle fibers from xenopus laevis. *J. Physiol.* 433: 307-326, 1991.
3. Westerblad H & DG Allen. Changes of myoplasmic calcium concentration during fatigue in single mouse muscle fibers. *J. Gen. Physiol.* 98: 615-635, 1991.

A.J. Baker, M.C. Longuemare, R. Brandes, M.W. Weiner and R.G. Miller

Muscle metabolism during fatiguing exercise

A. de Haan

Department of Muscle and Exercise Physiology, Faculty of Human Movement Sciences, Vrije Universiteit, Meibergdreef 15, 1105 AZ Amsterdam, The Netherlands.

Abstract In humans after short-term maximal exercise muscle glycogen levels are reduced to 75-80% of the initial muscle content. However, data obtained from maximally activated rat muscles show that after only a few seconds of exercise total glycogen depletion had occurred in many fast fibres. It is argued that during short maximal exercise, effects of glycogen depletion in some fibres may lead to the inability to sustain the required high level of exercise. During short maximal exercise and at the end of prolonged heavy exercise large amounts of IMP and ammonia are produced. In experiments with rat muscles it was found that the extent of loss of force (and power) at the end of all kinds of exercise, was related to the amount of IMP produced. It is suggested that the IMP produced may help to control the energy flux through the muscle cells by inhibiting contractile function and thus protect the muscle against an energy crisis. The high rate of production of IMP by muscles which are glycogen depleted indicate that IMP might be a linkage between glycogen depletion and fatigue.

Glycogen and endurance

In the late 1960's several reports by Scandinavian investigators showed that glycogen stored in skeletal muscles was a major determinant for endurance of long-term heavy exercise. First it was shown that performance time was linearly related to the amount of stored glycogen in the muscle before exercise (Ahlborg et al. 1967). In a subsequent paper it was demonstrated that work time was affected by manipulation of the amount of glycogen storage by different diets (Bergström et al. 1967). The conclusion from these papers, i.e. that glycogen was a limiting factor for performance of long-term heavy exercise, was universally accepted and used by endurance athletes to improve performance by different "carbohydrate loading" regimes.

In contrast to long-term exercise, relatively high muscle glycogen levels were found after fatiguing short-term high-intensity exercise (e.g. Boobis et al. 1983, Sahlin et al. 1975, 1976, 1989). It has further been demonstrated that human high-intensity exercise performance was not impaired by low muscle glycogen concentrations (varying from 153 to 426 μmol glucose units/g^{dw}; Symons & Jacobs, 1989). Also the rate of glycogenolysis during short-term tetanic stimulation of rat muscles was not affected by glycogen levels between 80 and 165 μmol/g^{dw}; Spriet et al. 1990). Based on these data glycogen depletion seems to play a non-significant role in fatigue during short-term high-intensity exercise. However, all these data were obtained from whole muscle samples. During high-intensity exercise it is necessary to recruit almost all the muscle fibres (e.g. Vøllestad et al., 1985). Reduction in muscle performance may occur by fatigue of all fibres, but it is more rational to expect a selective fatigue of some muscle fibres which have a low resistance against fatigue. Since almost all fibres are active, fatigue of only a few fibres will already result in a decrease of performance, with only little effect on whole muscle metabolism. Therefore it is necessary to investigate metabolic changes in different fibre populations of muscles.

In order to investigate changes in glycogen levels in different fibre types, histochemical techniques for fibre typing and substrate staining were used. The periodic acid-Shiff (PAS) stain is specific for glycogen (see e.g. Vøllestad et al. 1984) and is used for detection of glycogen depletion in fibre types and in individual muscle fibres. Using these techniques, it was shown that during long-term exercise the slow-oxidative fibres were depleted first, followed by the fast-oxidative and finally the fast-glycolytic fibres in man (Gollnick et al. 1973) and rat (Armstrong et al. 1974). In contrast, these reports showed that during high intensity exercise, fast-glycolytic fibres started to use glycogen immediately at the start of exercise.

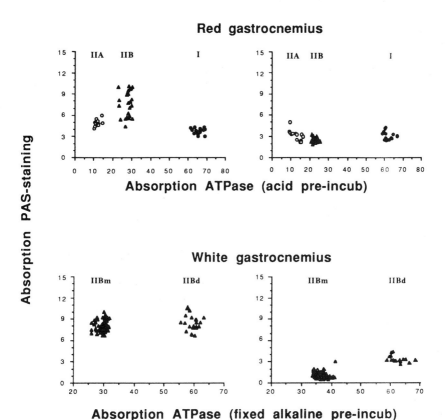

Figure 1. Example of changes in PAS-absorption in different fibre types in red and white rat medial gastrocnemius muscles.

The experimental muscle was maximally stimulated to perform 40 successive dynamic contractions within 10s (see group C in Fig. 3). The controls were resting contralateral muscles. The fibres were classified according to Lind & Kernell (1991). The absorption data are given in arbitrary units. These experiments were performed in collaboration with A.Lind and D.Kernell of the Department of Neurophysiology, University of Amsterdam, The Netherlands.

In a recent study we investigated glycogen degradation in fibres of in situ medial gastrocnemius muscles. These muscles of anaesthetized rats were maximally stimulated (1mA; 120Hz) at a temperature of 36°C using an isovelocity measuring device (de Haan et al. 1989). The muscles performed 40 dynamic contractions (duration 84ms) within 10s. During the 10s exercise (total active duration: 3.4s) work output per contraction decreased to <10% of the output in the first contraction (see group C in Fig. 3). At the end of the exercise the muscles were frozen in isopentane pre-cooled in liquid nitrogen. 10μm sections were cut from the midsection of the muscles and stained for fibre typing and PAS. Identification of fibre types I, IIA, IIBd and IIBm occurred as described by Lind & Kernell (1991) by a combination of ATPase stainings after an acid pre-incubation (Brooke & Kaiser, 1970) and after a fixed alkaline pre-incubation (Guth & Samaha, 1970).

Figure 1 presents examples of PAS absorption measurements of fibres in resting and exercised muscles. In the red portion of the gastrocnemius muscle all 4 fibre types are present, while in the white portion of the muscle only types IIBd and IIBm are seen (Fig. 1). Although all fibres were maximally stimulated, glycogen utilization (as judged by the change in PAS absorption) was most pronounced in the type IIBm fibres and hardly any changes in PAS absorption occurred in the type I fibres. These data show that in rats severe glycogen depletion of fast fibres can occur in short duration maximal exercise of only a few seconds. Differences exist between rats and humans with respect to total content of glycogen and possibly in maximal rates of glycogen degradation. Nevertheless, effects resulting from glycogen depletion may play also a role in fatigue during short-term high-intensity exercise in humans. This is supported by the observations of Gollnick et al. (1974) who showed that after the first exercise bout (3min at 120% VO_{2max}) some FT fibres were already glycogen depleted.

Glycogen depletion patterns and motor unit recruitment

The data in Fig. 1 show that the absence of a change in PAS-absorption in slow fibres (Type I) does not necessarily mean that these fibres were not active during exercise, because in this preparation all fibres were maximally activated. Thus although during high-intensity exercise in humans only little evidence of glycogen oxidation is seen in the slow-twitch fibres (Gollnick et al. 1973), one cannot conclude that those fibres had not been active during this type of exercise. Clearly care is needed in interpreting glycogen depletion patterns in terms of fibre activity (and fibre recruitment). The relation between glycogen depletion patterns and fibre activity may also be disturbed by the existence of differences between fibres with respect to the possibilities of utilizing other substrates (like free-fatty acids and amino acids) as well as glycogen for ATP generation. Moreover, some reports suggest that also non-exercising muscles in the rat may utilize glycogen at a similar rate as the exercising muscles (McDermott et al. 1987, Bonen 1989). In these studies comparison was made between the changes in glycogen levels of rat hindlimb muscles after treadmill exercise with and without hindlimb suspension. All types of muscle (white gastrocnemius as well as soleus muscle) showed similar glycogen degradations irrespective of their activity. They further showed that the loss of glycogen in the non-exercising muscles was dependent on the increase in the plasma epinephrine concentration (McDermott et al. 1987). This dependency on epinephrine is in agreement with earlier reports from Gorski et al. (1978) and Richter et al. (1981, 1982). They suggested that the first enhancement of glycogen utilization during exercise is induced by the onset of contractile activity, but that later in the exercise epinephrine is necessary to maintain an enhanced rate of degradation. The findings that muscles which had not been activated also showed glycogen degradation further demonstrates, that one should be careful with using glycogen depletion patterns to study motor-unit recruitment patterns during exercise.

Glycogen depletion and fatigue: why?

In spite of the enormous attention given to glycogen oxidation and fatigue, it remains unclear why low glycogen levels results in fatigue. The most popular theory on why glycogen is necessary for ATP production is the anaplerotic theory (Conlee 1987). According to this theory glycogen oxidation provides pyruvate, which can be used for reactions to supply intermediates of the tricarboxylic acid (TCA) cycle. Oxaloacetate can be formed by carboxylation of pyruvate (by pyruvate carboxykinase) and of phosphoenolpyruvate (PEP; by PEP carboxykinase). α-Ketoglutarate can be formed by the aminotransferase reaction, where pyruvate is converted to alanine at the expense of glutamate (by Glutamate-Pyruvate Transaminase). During short-term high-intensity exercise (Essén & Kayser 1978) and during the first minutes of prolonged exercise there is an increase in the amount of TCA cycle intermediates (TCAI; Sahlin et al. 1990). An increase in TCAI is needed to obtain a high flux through the cycle, which is necessary to feed the mitochondria with reduction equivalents (NADH) for the respiratory chain. During prolonged exercise a decrease of TCAI is observed (Sahlin et al. 1990).

It has been suggested that degradation of branched-chain amino acids (BCAA) is one of the major reactions which leads to draining of intermediates from the TCA cycle (Wagenmakers et al. 1991). Through activation of the branched-chain 2-oxo acid dehydrogenase complex, BCAA are converted to 2-oxo acids, while α-ketogluterate is aminated to glutamate. Glutamate

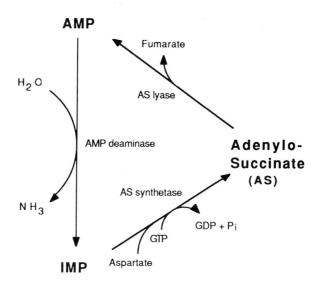

AMP

Fumarate

H$_2$O

AS lyase

AMP deaminase

**Adenylo-
Succinate
(AS)**

AS synthetase

GDP + P$_i$

NH$_3$

GTP

IMP Aspartate

Figure 2. The Purine Nucleotide Cycle (Lowenstein 1972).

can then be used to form glutamine or alanine (by the Glutamate Pyruvate Transaminase reaction). The release of glutamine and alanine from the muscles during prolonged exercise (Sahlin et al. 1990) indicate that draining of TCAI occurs. Thus, in order to maintain a high flux through the TCA cycle it is necessary to remain supplying the TCA cycle with intermediates. It has been suggested that when muscle glycogen is depleted, the supply of pyruvate will be reduced leading to a limitation of anaplerotic reactions. Because of the resulting decrease in maximal rate of ATP production transient increases in ADP and AMP will occur, which will then lead to contractile failure (Sahlin et al. 1990).

Purine Nucleotide Cycle and fatigue

It was further argued that the occurrence of transient increases in ADP and AMP was supported by the observed increases in inosine-5'-monophosphate (IMP) and ammonia, because ADP and AMP are both activators of the enzyme AMP-deaminase (Sahlin et al. 1990). This reaction is part of the purine nucleotide cycle (PNC; Fig. 2; Lowenstein 1972), which cycle is active during exercise (Aragon & Lowenstein 1980). There are several functions suggested for the PNC (Tullson & Terjung 1989; Lowenstein 1972, 1990):

1. During one complete cycle one aspartate is deaminated to fumarate. Thus the cycle can provide TCAI from amino acid sources and thus support the replenishment of TCA cycle intermediates. Because of the relatively low activities of the enzymes for reamination of IMP to AMP this replenishment probably does not occur during short maximal exercise.

In the other suggested functions only the AMP deaminase reaction is involved.
2. One of the main functions is thought to be the control of relative concentrations of ATP, ADP and AMP. The maintenance of a relatively high ATP/ADP ratio (and phosphorylation potential) is important for many cellular reactions.
3. Produced NH$_3$ may take up H$^+$-ions and thus serve as a pH-buffer. NH$_3$ is also an activator of phosphofructokinase and hence glycolysis.
4. Produced IMP may stimulate glycogen degradation by activation of the enzyme phosphorylase b.

A. de Haan

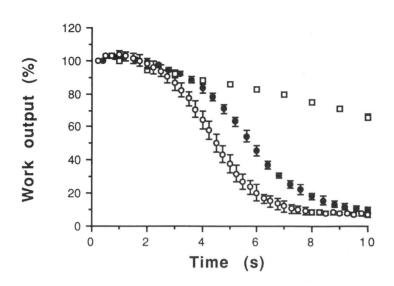

Figure 3. Changes in work output (mean ± SD) during exercise.
Rat medial gastrocnemius muscles were maximally stimulated to perform a series of contractions within 10s.
Group A (..): 10 contractions (duration 342ms shortening velocity (v) 80mm/s).
Group B (o): 25 contractions (duration 134ms: v=50mm/s).
Group C (o): 40 contractions (duration 84ms: v=80mm/s).
Total stimulation time was ~3.4s in all groups. Shortening distance was 6mm (~17% of the muscle belly length). (Data from de Haan, 1990).

All these suggested functions will help to preserve a high rate of ATP production in order to sustain the exercise. For living cells it is important to control the energy flux and thus to maintain a balance between ATP producing and ATP utilizing processes. Occurrence of an imbalance may result in loss of main cell functions and necrosis. Therefore muscle cells should not only control ATP producing reactions but should also control ATP utilizing processes (as contractile activity).

It has been suggested that the production of IMP may play a role in the control of contractile activity and thus serve as a protecting mechanism (Berden et al. 1986; Westra et al. 1986). It has been shown that the loss of force during one continuous or during series of repeated isometric or dynamic contractions co-incided with an increase in muscle IMP content (Westra et al. 1986; de Haan et al. 1988, 1991). In recent experiments different protocols of short-term high-intensity exercise of rat medial gastrocnemius muscles lead to different extents of loss of performance (Fig. 3). In groups A, B and C the muscles performed 10, 25 and 40 contractions within 10s with shortening velocities of 20, 50 and 80mm/s, respectively.

Total stimulation time during the 10s exercise was 3.4s in all protocols. Whereas ~90% of the initial work output was lost at the end of the exercise in groups B and C, the loss of work output was only ~35% in group A (Fig. 3). Muscle phosphocreatine and lactate concentrations at the end of exercise were similar for the 3 groups (Table 1). However, reductions in ATP and concommitant productions of IMP were higher for the 2 groups with the greatest loss of performance. The very high IMP concentrations after exercise in group C correspond with the large depletion of glycogen found at the end of this exercise (Fig. 1). Formation of IMP and NH_3 in glycogen depleted muscles and fibres have also been reported for human muscles (Norman et al. 1988; Spencer et al. 1991; Broberg & Sahlin 1989).

Muscle metabolism during fatiguing exercise

Table 2. Metabolite concentrations of resting muscles (Control) and of muscles sampled after the 10s exercise period of the 3 different groups. (Data from de Haan, 1990)

	Control (n=18)	Group A (n=6)	Group B (n=6)	Group C (n=6)
PC	100.6 (4.7)	37.6 (5.1)	31.2 (7.2)	33.8 (7.5)
ATP	29.7 (2.3)	20.1 (2.2)	11.0 (1.2)	11.6 (1.2)
ADP	4.3 (0.2)	5.0 (0.2)	4.0 (0.7)	4.3 (0.3)
IMP	<1	9.9 (2.1)	18.6 (1.2)	17.8 (1.7)
Lactate	8.4 (2.4)	54.6 (10.1)	56.7 (5.1)	57.2 (6.5)

Mean data (SD) are given in µmol/gdw

It can be hypothetized therefore that severe depletion of glycogen would result in an increased formation of IMP, which compound would inhibit contractile activity. This hypothesis is supported by recent in vitro experiments which showed that IMP inhibits actin-stimulated myosin ATPase activity (Westra et al. 1992).

In conclusion, it is suggested that effects of glycogen depletion may play a role in fatigue during short-duration high-intensity exercise. Further, it is suggested that depletion of glycogen may lead to increased IMP levels, which would inhibit contractile function and thus lead to fatigue.

References

Ahlborg B, Bergström J, Ekelund, G and Hultman E (1967). Muscle glycogen and muscle electrolytes during prolonged physical exercise. *Acta Physiologica Scandinavia* **70**: 129-142

Aragón JJ & Lowenstein JM (1980). The purine nucleotide cycle. Comparison of the levels of citric acid cycle intermediates with the operation of the purine nucleotide cycle in rat muscle during exercise and recovery from exercise. *European Journal of Biochemistry* **110**: 371-177.

Armstrong RB, Saubert CW, Sembrowich WL, Shepherd RE and Gollnick PD (1974). Glycogen depletion in rat skeletal muscle fibers at different intensities and durations of exercise. *Pflügers Archiv* **352**: 243-256.

Berden JA, de Haan A, de Haan EJ, van Doorn JE, Hartog AF and Westra HG (1986). Has IMP a regulatory role during fatiguing contraction? IMP-binding sites on the myosin complex of rat muscle. *Journal of Physiology* **381**: 85P.

Bergström J, Hermansen L, Hultman E and Saltin B (1967). Diet, muscle glycogen and physical performance. *Acta Physiologica Scandinavia* **71**: 140-150.

Bonen A, McDermott JC and Hutber CA (1989). Carbohydrate metabolism in skeletal muscle: an update of current concepts. *International Journal of Sports Medicine* **10**: 385-401.

Boobis LH, Williams C and Wootton SA (1983). Human muscle metabolism during brief maximal exercise. *Journal of Physiology* **338**: 21-22P.

Broberg S & Sahlin K (1989). Adenine nucleotide degradation in human skeletal muscle during prolonged exercise. *Journal of Applied Physiology* **67**: 116-122.

Brooke MH & Kaiser KK (1970). Muscle fiber types: How many of what kind? *Archives Neurology* **23**: 369-379.

Conlee RK (1987). Muscle glycogen and exercise endurance: A twenty-year perspective. *Exercise and Sports Sciences Reviews* **15**: 1-29.

de Haan A, van Doorn JE and Sargeant AJ (1988). Age-related changes in power output during repetitive contractions of rat medial gastrocnemius muscle. *Pflügers Archiv* **412**: 665-667.

de Haan A, Jones DA and Sargeant AJ (1989). Changes in velocity of shortening, power output and relaxation rate during fatigue of rat medial gastrocnemius muscle. *Pflügers Archiv* **413**: 422-428.

de Haan A (1990). High-energy phosphates and fatigue during repeated dynamic contractions of rat muscle. *Experimental Physiology* **75**, 851-854.

de Haan A, de Ruiter CJ and Sargeant AJ (1991). Influence of age on fatigue, IMP production and efficiency. Abstract: Proceedings of the 8th International Biochemistry of Exercise Conference, Nagoya, Japan

Essén B & Kayser L (1978). Regulation of glycolysis in intermittent exercise in man. *Journal of Physiology* **281**: 499-511.

Gollnick PD, Piehl K and Saltin B (1974). Selective glycogen depletion patterns in human muscle fibres after exercise of varying intensity and at varying pedalling rates. *Journal of Physiology* **241**: 45-57.

Gollnick PD, Armstrong RB, Sembrowich WL, Shepherd RE and Saltin B (1973). Glycogen depletion patterns in human skeletal muscle fibers after heavy exercise. *Journal of Applied Physiology* **34** : 615-618.

Górski J (1978). Exercise-induced changes of reactivity of different types of muscle on glycogenolytic effect of adrenaline. *Pflügers Archiv* **373**: 1-7.

Guth L & Samaha FJ (1970). Procedure for the histochemical demonstration of actomyosin ATPase. Research note. *Experimental Neurology* **28**: 365-367.

Lind A & Kernell D (1991). Myofibrillar ATPase histochemistry of rat skeletal muscles: a two-dimensional quantitative approach. *The Journal of Histochemistry and Cytochemistry* **39**: 589-597.

Lowenstein JM (1972). Ammonia production in muscle and other tissues: the purine nucleotide cycle. *Physiological Reviews* **52**: 382-414.

Lowenstein JM (1990). The purine nucleotide cycle revised. *International Journal of Sports Medicine* **11** (suppl. 2): S37-S46.

McDermott JC, Elder GCB and Bonen A (1987). Adrenal hormones enhance glycogenolysis in non-exercising muscle during exercise. *Journal of Applied Physiology* **63**: 1275-1283.

Norman B, Sollevi A and Jansson E (1988). Increased IMP content in glycogen-depleted muscle fibres during submaximal exercise in man. *Acta Physiologica Scandinavia* **133**: 97-100.

Richter EA, Ruderman NB, Gravas H, Belur ER and Galbo H (1982). Muscle glycogenolysis during exercise: dual control by epinephrine and contractions. *American Journal of Physiology* **242**: E25-E32.

Richter EA , Galbo H and Christensen NJ (1981). Control of exercise-induced muscular glycogenolysis by adrenal medullary hormones in rats. *Journal of Applied Physiology* **50**: 21-26.

Sahlin K, Broberg S and Ren JM (1989). Formation of IMP in human skeletal muscle during incremental dynamic exercise. *Acta Physiologica Scandinavia* **136**: 193-198.

Sahlin K, Harris RC and Hultman E (1975). Creatine kinase equilibrium and lactate content compared with muscle pH in tissue samples obtained after isometric exercise. *Biochemical Journal* **152**: 173-180.

Sahlin K, Harris RC, Nylind B and Hultman E (1976). Lactate content and pH in muscle samples obtained after dynamic exercise. *Pflügers Archiv* **367**: 143-149.

Sahlin K, Katz A and Broberg S (1990). Tricarboxylic acid cycle intermediates in human muscle during prolonged exercise. *American Journal of Physiology* **259**: C834-C841.

Spencer MK, Yan Z and Katz A (1991). Carbohydrate supplementation attenuates IMP formation in human muscle during prolonged exercise. *American Journal of Physiology* **261**: C71-C76.

Spriet LL, Berardinucci L, Marsh DR, Campell CB and Graham TE (1990). Glycogen content has no effect on skeletal muscle glycogenolysis during short-term tetanic stimulation. *Journal of Applied Physiology* **68**: 1883-1888.

Symons JD & Jacobs I (1989). High-intensity exercise performance is not impaired by low intramuscular glycogen. *Medicine and Science in Sports and Exercise:* **21**: 550-557.

Tullson PC & Terjung RL (1991). Adenine nucleotide metabolism in contracting skeletal muscle. *Exercise and Sports Sciences Reviews* **19**, 507-538.

Vøllestad NK, Vaage O and Hermansen L (1984). Muscle glycogen depletion patterns in type I and subgroups of type II fibres during prolonged severe exercise in man. *Acta Physiologica Scandinavia* **122**: 433-441.

Vøllestad NK & Blom PCS (1985). Effect of varying exercise intensity on glycogen depletion in human muscle fibres. *Acta Physiologica Scandinavia* **125**: 395, 405.

Wagenmakers AJM, Beckers EJ, Brouns F, Kuipers H, Soeters PB, van der Vusse GJ and Saris WHM (1991). Carbohydrate supplemention, glycogen depletion, and amino acid metabolism during exercise. *American Journal of Physiology* **260**: E883-E890.

Westra HG, de Haan A, van Doorn JE and de Haan EJ (1986). IMP production and energy metabolism during exercise in rats in relation to age. *Biochemical Journal* **239**: 751-755.

Westra HG, Berden JA and Pasman WJ (1992). A model for regulation of actin activated myosin ATPase inhibition of the formation of actin-myosin complex. In: Sargeant AJ & Kernell D (Eds). Neuromuscular Fatigue. Royal Netherlands Academy of Sciences - Elsevier Biomedical BV, Amsterdam, The Netherlands.

A model for the regulation of actin-activated Mg^{2+}-myosin ATPase activity: inhibition of the formation of actin-myosin complex by IMP

H.G. Westra, J.A. Berden[*] and W.J. Pasman

Dept. of Muscle and Exercise Physiology, Faculty of Human Movement Sciences, Vrije Universiteit, Meibergdreef 15; 1105 AZ Amsterdam, The Netherlands, [*] E.C. Slater Institute for Biochemical Resarch, University of Amsterdam.

One of the topics in our research program is the study of the metabolic events during muscular contraction under anaerobic conditions. We suggest that the decrease in force or power output during exhaustive exercise might at least in part occur because of a metabolic down regulation of the acto-myosin ATPase activity due to IMP formation.

During contraction ATP is converted to ADP. Figure 1 summarizes the pathways for resynthesis of ATP from ADP. In one of the reactions, the adenylate kinase reaction, AMP is formed which can be deaminated to IMP and ammonia by AMP deaminase. In previous experiments with the rat fast-twitch quadriceps muscle we found that during a maximal continuous isometric contraction (15 s) about 6 µmol IMP.g dry weight $^{-1}$ was formed (Westra et al., 1989). After several repeated contractions we found higher total energy-rich phosphate consumption as well as higher IMP formation (Westra et al., 1986, 1989). During exhaustive dynamic contractions even higher IMP concentrations were found (de Haan et al., 1988, 1990).There are several speculations about the possible function of AMP deaminase. In

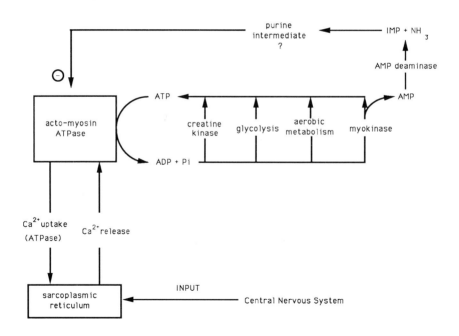

Fig.1. A model for regulation of acto-myosine ATPase during exhaustive contractions

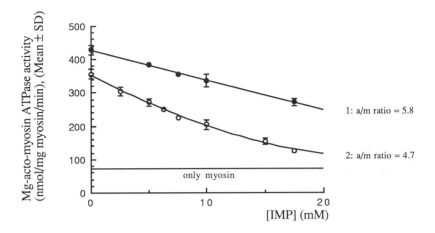

Fig.2. The inhibitory effect of IMP on Mg^{2+}-myosin ATPase activity and actin-activated Mg^{2+}-myosin ATPase activity. The Mg^{2+}-myosin ATPase activity (70 nmol.mg protein^{-1}.min^{-1} is independent of IMP
For curve 1: $v = 427 - 9.0$ [IMP]; $r = 0.998$
For curve 2: $v = 354 - 18.8$ [IMP] $+ 0.34$ [IMP]^2; $r = 0.996$

general the enzyme is thought to play a regulatory role in stimulating ATP *synthesis* (Sugdon and Newsholme, 1975; Aragon et al., 1980) and to keep the relative nucleotide concentrations optimal for contraction (Lowenstein, 1972). Moreover we think that IMP plays a key-role in the regulation of ATP *consumption*. Experiments carried out by our group during isometric (Berden at al., 1986; Westra et al., 1989) and dynamic contractions (de Haan et al., 1990) with fast-twitch rat muscles suggest that IMP formation is dependent on the stress laid upon the muscle and that the production of IMP could be a signal to the muscle cell that contractions were carried out under exhaustive conditions.

This conclusion brought us to the following idea. For the muscle functioning **in vivo** it is necessary to be able to relax. For relaxation ATP must be available to reabsorb the calcium into the sarcoplasmic reticulum and to break down the actomyosin complex.As stimulation from the central nervous system and the intracellular metabolism are two more or less independent phenomena the muscle cell should have a mechanism which regulates the balance between the rate of ATP consumption and the rate of ATP synthesis, in order to protect itself against too low ATP concentrations which might result in an unability to relax. From these observations we formulated the following working *hypothesis*:

Previous to an "energy crisis" in the muscle cell, the contractile mechanism is switched off in order to save energy for relaxation and to economize remaining energy for the maintenance of cell integrity (see figure 1). The down regulation of the contractile machinery might be caused by IMP, formed during exhaustive contractions.

To test this hypothesis we carried out experiments with isolated actin and myosin from rabbit fast-twitch muscles. Measurements of Mg^{2+}-myosin ATPase activity and actin-activated Mg^{2+}-myosin ATPase activity were carried out in the absence and presence of variable concentrations of IMP and AMP under the following standard conditions: 25 mM TRIS (pH 7.0), 40 mM KCl, 10 mM $MgCl_2$, 2.5 mM ATP and an ATP regenerating system. The myosin concentration was 51 nM and the actin concentration either 240 nM or 300 nM (actin/myosin ratio of 4.7 and 5.8, respectively).

The results of the experiments in the presence of IMP (shown in figure 2) are the following:
1. IMP did not inhibit the Mg^{2+}-myosin ATPase activity.

2. IMP inhibits the actin-activated Mg^{2+}-myosin ATPase activity. The degree of inhibition depends on the actin/myosin ratio; at higher ratios the inhibition is less.

AMP had similar effects (not shown) to IMP. However, the physiological significance is probably less than that of IMP because the AMP concentration hardly changes during exhaustive exercise from the resting value of about 0.1 mM, whereas the IMP concentration can increase up to 5 mM.

Since IMP does not inhibit pure Mg^{2+}-myosin ATPase activity, we suggest that IMP prevents the formation of actin-myosin complexes. The overall consequence of an inhibition by IMP would be:

1. decrease of cross-bridge formation leading to a decrease in mechanical output
2. prevention of contracture development during an "energy crisis" (relaxation is favored).
3. The cell can economize remaining energy for the maintenance of membrane integrity and interior milieu for temporal survival.

References

Aragon, JJ , Tornheim, K and Lowenstein JM (1980). On a possible role of IMP in the regulation of phosphorylase activity in skeletal muscle. *Febs Letters* **117**; K 56-64.

Berden, JA, de Haan A, de Haan EJ, van Doorn EJ, Hartog AF, Westra HG (1986) Has IMP a regulatory role during fatiguing contraction? IMP-binding sites on the myosin complex of rat muscle. *Journal of Physiology* **381**, 85P.

de Haan A, van Doorn JE and Sargeant AJ (1988). Age-related changes in power output during repetitive contractions of rat medial gastrocnemius muscle. *Pflügers Archiv* **412**; 665-667.

de Haan A (1990). High-energy phosphates and fatigue during repeated dynamic contractions of rat muscle. *Experimental Physiology* **75**, 851-854

Lowenstein JM (1972). Ammonia production in muscle and other tissue: the purine nucleotide cycle. *Physiological Reviews* **52**; 382-414.

Sugden, PH and Newsholm, EA (1975). The effects of ammonium, inorganic phosphate and potassium ions on the activity of phosphofructokinase from muscle and nervous tissues of vertebrates and invertebrates. *Biochemical Journal* **150**; 113-122.

Westra, HG, de Haan, A, van Doorn JE and de Haan EJ (1986) IMP production and energy metabolism during exercise in rats in relation to age. *Biochemical Journal* **239**, 751-755.

Westra, HG, de Haan, A, van Doorn JE and de Haan EJ (1989) Anaerobic chemical changes and mechanical output during isometric tetani of rat muscle in situ. *Pflügers Archiv*, **412**, 121 - 127.

Skeletal muscle energy metabolism and fatigue during intense contraction in man

Paul Greenhaff*, Karin Söderlund** and Eric Hultman

Dept. Clinical Chemistry II, Huddinge University Hospital, Karolinska Institute, S-141 86 Huddinge, Sweden.
*present address Dept. Physiology & Pharmacology, Queens Medical Centre, University Nottingham, Nottingham NG7 2UH, UK.
**present address Dept. Physiology III, Karolinska Institute, Box 5626, 114 86 Stockholm, Sweden.

The rate of skeletal muscle anaerobic ATP resynthesis is rapid when compared with aerobic resynthesis, however a high rate of anaerobic resynthesis can only be maintained for short periods of time. Table 1 shows the rates of ATP resynthesis from phosphocreatine (PCr) and glycolysis during 30s of near maximal isometric contraction in man. After only 1.3s of contraction the rate of PCr utilisation begins to decline, while the corresponding rate from glycolysis does not peak until after 3s of contraction This suggests that the rapid initial utilisation of PCr may buffer the momentary lag in energy provision from glycolysis. There is also a progressive decline in ATP provision from both substrates after their initial peaks e.g. the rates of ATP provision from PCr and glycolysis during the final 10s of contraction amount to 2 and 40%, respectively of their respective peak rates of production. Similar findings, involving isokinetic and dynamic exercise, have been reported by other research groups (Boobis et al. 1982, Jones et al. 1985). Interestingly, in all of these studies, in conjunction with the decline in anaerobic ATP production was a decline in force production and power output. It is tempting to postulate therefore, that the development of fatigue was attributable to the decline in ATP provision. Alternatively however, the decline in energy provision may simply be a function of a decline in the rate of ATP utilisation which will accompany any decline in force production.

Table 1. Rates of anaerobic ATP resynthesis from phosphocreatine (PCr) degradation and glycolysis during intense contraction in man. Values were calculated from muscle metabolite changes measured in muscle biopsy samples obtained during intense intermittent electrically evoked (50Hz) isometric contraction (Hultman and Sjöholm 1983, Hultman et al. 1990).

	ATP production (mmol/kg dm/s) from:	
Duration (s)	PCr	glycolysis
0-1.3	9.0	2.0
0-2.6	7.5	4.3
0-5	5.3	4.4
0-10	4.2	4.5
10-20	2.2	4.5
20-30	0.2	2.1

The values shown in table 1 were calculated from the metabolite changes measured in muscle biopsy samples obtained from the quadriceps femoris muscle of normal healthy volunteers. However, it is known that human skeletal muscle is composed of at least two functionally and metabolically different fibre types. Type I fibres have been shown to have a high aerobic capacity, to be slow contracting with a low power output and to be fatigue resistant. Conversely, type II fibres have a high anaerobic capacity, are fast contracting with a high peak power output and fatigue rapidly (for comprehensive review see Green 1986). Evidence from animal studies performed on muscles composed of predominantly type I or type II fibres (Barany 1967, Hintz et al. 1982) and from one study performed using bundles of similar human muscle fibre types (Faulkner et al. 1986), suggest that the rapid marked rise and subsequent decline in maximal power output observed during intense muscle contraction in man may be closely related to activation and rapid fatigue of type II fibres during contraction.

Recently we have attempted to relate the decline in whole muscle force production during intense contraction in man to the metabolic changes occurring in individual muscle fibre types (Greenhaff et al. 1991, Hultman et al. 1991, Söderlund et al. 1992). These studies have involved individual muscle fibre fragments being dissected from biopsy samples and, after fibre type characterisation, being used to determine single fibre ATP, PCr and glycogen concentrations. The latter study involved muscle biopsy samples being obtained from the quadriceps muscle group before and after 10 and 20s of intense isometric contraction, induced by intermittent percutaneous electrical stimulation (50Hz; 1.6s stimulation, 1.6s rest). During the initial 10s of stimulation, the rates of PCr utilisation in type I and II fibres were 3.3 and 5.3 mmol/kg dm/s, respectively. During the subsequent 10s of stimulation, the rate of PCr utilisation in type I fibres remained fairly constant, declining by ~15%. However, the corresponding rate in type II fibres declined by ~60% and, at the end of the stimulation period, the PCr store of this fibre type was close to zero.

The rate of glycogen utilisation over the 20s stimulation period in type II fibres (6.3 mmol/kg dm/s) was rapid when compared to the negligible rate observed in type I fibres (0.6 mmol/kg dm/s), and was in excess of both the measured and calculated maximal rates of glycogen utilisation determined for mixed fibred muscle. Unfortunately, the rate of single fibre glycogen utilisation was not determined for the initial 10s of contraction, therefore it is not possible to determine whether the decline in glycogenolysis observed in mixed fibred muscle (Table 1) occurred solely in type II fibres. However, in an experiment where electrical stimulation was maintained for 30s (Greenhaff et al. 1991), the rate of glycogenolysis in type II fibres was 3.5 mmol/kg dm/s over the stimulation period, and the corresponding rate in type I fibres was 0.2 mmol/kg dm/s. It is plausible to suggest therefore that the observed decline in glycogen utilisation in mixed fibred muscle during intense electrical stimulation is probably restricted to type II fibres. The relatively low rate of ATP utilisation by type I fibres, together with their high capacity to resynthesise ATP aerobically, may explain the observed low rate of glycogen utilisation by these fibres during intense intermittent contraction. It is possible that the intermittent nature of the contraction (1.6s stimulation, 1.6s rest) may be important in dictating the oxygen availability to this fibre type.

In parallel with the decline in whole muscle force production during intense isometric contraction is a marked decline in the rates of PCr and glycogen utilisation in type II fibres. In the case of type I fibres, the corresponding rates of utilisation remain relatively unchanged. Evidence suggests that after ~20s of intense contraction the PCr store of type II fibres will be almost totally depleted and the rate of glycogen utilisation will be close to maximal or even on the decline in this fibre type. At this point, no alternative mechanisms will be available for type II fibres to maintain the required ATP resynthesis rate and compensate for the depleted PCr stores and declining, or soon to be declining, rate of glycogen utilisation. In short therefore, the declining rate of ATP resynthesis will be insufficient to maintain force production and fatigue will occur.

References

Barany M (1967). ATPase activity of myosin correlated with speed of muscle shortening. *Journal of General Physiology* **50** (suppl 2), 197-218.

Boobis LH, C Williams & SA Wooton (1982). Human muscle metabolism during brief maximal exercise in man. *Journal of Physiology (London)* **338**, 21-22P.

Faulkner JA, Claflin DR & McCully KK (1986). Power output of fast and slow fibres from human skeletal muscles. In: *Human Muscle Power*. Eds, Jones NL, McCartney N & McComas AJ, Human Kinetics Publ., Champaign, IL. pp81-89.

Green HJ (1986). Muscle power: Fibre type recruitment, metabolism and fatigue. In: *Human Muscle Power*. Eds, Jones NL, McCartney N & McComas AJ, Human Kinetics Publ., Champaign, IL. pp65-80.

Greenhaff PL, Ren J-M, Söderlund K & Hultman E (1991). Energy metabolism in single muscle fibres during contraction witout and with epinephrine infusion. *American Journal of Physiology* **260**, E713-E718.

Hintz CS, Chi MM-Y, Fell RD, Ivy JL, Kaiser KK, Lowry CV & Lowry OH (1982). Metabolite changes in individual rat muscle fibres during stimulation. *American Journal of Physiology* **242**, C218-C228.

Hultman E & Sjöholm H (1983). Substrate availability. In: *Biochemistry of Exercise, International Series on Sport Sciences*. Eds, Knuttgen HG, Vogel JA, & J Poortmans, **13**, Human Kinetics Publ., Champaign, IL. pp 63-75.

Hultman E, Bergstrom M, Spreit LL & Söderlund K (1990). Energy metabolism and fatigue. In: *Biochemistry of Exercise, International Series on Sport Sciences*. Eds, Taylor AW, Gollnick PD, Green HJ, Ianuzzo CD, Noble EG, Metivier G, & Sutton J, **21**, Human Kinetics Publ., Champaign, IL. pp 73-92.

Hultman E, Greenhaff PL, Ren J-M & Söderlund K (1991). Energy metabolism and fatigue during intense muscle contraction. *Biochemical Society Transactions* **19**, 347-353.

Jones NL, McCartney N, Graham T, Spriet LL, Kowalchuk JM, Haigenhauser GJF & Sutton JR (1985). Muscle performance and metabolism in maximal isokinetic cycling at slow and fast speeds. *Journal of Applied Physiology* **59**, 132-136.

Söderlund K, Greenhaff PL & Hultman E (1992). Energy metabolism in type I and type II human muscle fibres during short term electrical stimulation at different frequencies. *Acta Physiologica Scandinavica* **144**, 15-22.

Inter-relation of electro-mechanical coupling and chemistry in the study of fatigue by ^{31}P-NMR spectroscopy

H. Gibson & R.H.T. Edwards

Magnetic Resonance Research Centre and Muscle Research Centre, Department of Medicine, University of Liverpool, P.O. Box 147, Liverpool L69 3BX, UK

Introduction

The application of ^{31}P magnetic resonance spectrocopy (MRS) to the study of human muscle has helped to further our understanding of the metabolic processes of fatigue. Despite the ease of access to muscle and the use of simple surface coil techniques, small magnet bore size and the inability to electrically stimulate muscle within the magnet have previously limited the objective electrophysiological analysis of muscle during fatiguing activity. Using a large bore magnet, we have developed a system for the electrical stimulation and force recording of human quadriceps, a well studied muscle group by conventional laboratory techniques (e.g., Bergstrom & Hultman, 1991). This has permitted a novel approach to the analysis of the inter-relation of electro-mechanical coupling and chemistry during stimulated fatiguing activity and subsequent recovery. Preliminary results for a typical subject are presented below.

Methods

Subjects were placed lying supine on the bed of a 1.5T General Electric SIGNA 48cm whole body MR system with the legs placed over a wedge-shaped polystyrene foam block, such that the knee angle was 105°. A restraining strap was placed around the waist. Isometric force was obtained from a specially constructed strain gauge and attached to the ankle via an inextensible strap. Percutaneous stimulation was achieved by the use of two gel defibrillator pads (3M) placed over the proximal and distal portions of the thigh and strapped in place. Small copper foil plates (3cm sq) were used to pass current from the stimulation leads to the defrillator pads. ^{31}P spectra were obtained with pulse and acquire sequences as the average of two aquisitions at a repetition time of 12 seconds using a surface coils for signal sampling. The stimulator was triggered by a pulse programme on an Apple II computer, itself triggered by the magnets' computer. Tetanic contractions of up to 80% of the maximal voluntary contraction (MVC) were achieved.

Studies were carried out with fatigue produced under conditions of open or occluded circulation (using a sphygmomanometer placed around the thigh) by the methods used previously for the adductor pollicis muscle (Cooper et al., 1988). Activity consisted of 14 (occluded conditions) or 50 (non-occluded conditions) trains of programmed stimulation myograms (PSM) consisting of impulses delivered at 1, 10, 20, 50 and 100 Hz (1 sec each, 10 Hz for 2 secs). Recovery was monitored for up to 15 minutes.

Results

Both ischaemic and non-occluded regimes produced marked reductions in force at all frequencies of stimulation, although these were greater for the ischaemic contractions. Reduction of PCr was noted immediately on activity with a concommitant increase in Pi. Stoichiometry was preserved in all studies. In some subjects splitting of the Pi peak was observed. This was abolished by ischaemic activity, although broadening of the Pi peak was noted, reflecting the possible contribution of different fibre types populations with differing metabolic characteristics (Achten et al., 1990). In one study increasing stimulation voltage in order to ensure that the signal was obtained from fully activated muscle only (80% MVC) did not abolish Pi splitting, although it is difficult to ensure no contamination of the signal by incompletely stimulated muscle i.e., a partial volume effect.

The inter-relations of force, electro-mechanical coupling and energy status of muscle under conditions of free circulation and ischaemia are shown in Figure 1.

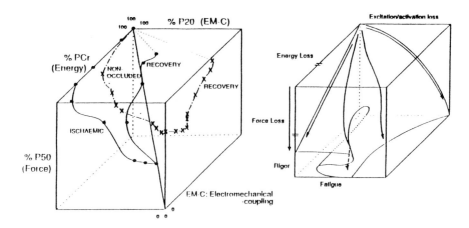

Figure 1: Three-dimensional plot based on the 'catastrophe theory' representation (inset) of inter-relations between force (stimulated tetanic force at 50Hz, P50), energy (as represented by phosphoryl creatine, PCr) and electro-mechanical coupling (represented by the force at 20Hz, P20) for ischaemic and non-occluded contractions.

Discussion

The combination of MRS and electrophysiological measurements undertaken in this study has enabled us to visualise in a three-dimensional model the relative importance of the possible mechanisms contributing to fatigue (Figure 1). It can be clearly seen from this model that fatigue and recovery under non-occluded conditions and ischaemia follow different pathways. Moreover, fatigue and recovery curves differ., i.e. hysteresis occurs. Using these techniques it may be possible to model all forms of activity, including stimulated, voluntary and submaximal exercise, permitting a greater understanding of the complex integration of processes contributing to muscle fatigue.

References

Achten E, Cauteren M van, Willem R, Luypaert R, Malaisse WJ, Bosch G van., Delanghe G, Meirleir K. de & Osteaux M (1990). 31P-NMR spectroscopy and the metabolic properties of different muscle fibres. *Journal of Applied Physiology* **68**,644-649.

Bergstrom M & Hultman E (1991) Relaxation and force during fatigue and recovery of the human quadriceps muscle: relations to metabolite changes. *Pflügers Archives* **418**, 153-160.

Cooper RG, Gibson H, Stokes MJ & Edwards RHT (1988) Human muscle fatigue: frequency dependence of excitation and force generation. *Journal of Physiology* **397**,585-599.

Section II

EMG related processes

The role of the Na^+,K^+-pump in delaying muscle fatigue

A.J. McComas, V. Galea, R.W. Einhorn, A.L. Hicks & S. Kuiack

Departments of Biomedical Sciences and Medicine, McMaster University, Health Sciences Centre, Hamilton, Ontario Canada L8N 3Z5

Abstract Through increased electrogenic activity, the Na^+,K^+-pump can maintain, or even increase, muscle fibre membrane potentials during muscle contractions, and can thereby compensate for the rise in interstitial K^+ concentration. During submaximal contractions the enhanced pumping affects quiescent fibres as well as the contracting ones. In human subjects the pump effects can be detected by changes in the muscle compound action potential. Intramuscular release of noradrenaline is probably one of the factors stimulating the pump.

There has long been speculation that K^+, released into the interstitial spaces by contracting muscle fibres, might contribute to muscle fatigue by blocking impulse conduction (e.g. Sjøgaard 1990). Two types of experiment would appear to support this proposition. One has been the use of ion-sensitive electrodes to demonstrate substantial elevations in interstitial K^+ concentration in contracting muscles (see below). The other approach has been to bathe isolated muscles in solutions containing raised K^+ concentrations and to show reductions in muscle compound action potentials or force (Jones 1981; Clausen & Everts 1991). In this paper we shall argue a contrary view by showing that, although $[K^+]$ is indeed raised in the interstitial spaces, it does not contribute to the decline in force at physiological rates of muscle excitation, because of the powerful intervention of the electrogenic Na^+,K^+-pump. Rather it appears that the pump is able to maintain the excitability of the muscle fibre plasmalemma and to ensure that the surface action potential retains its full size, until force has started to decline. In developing this proposition, the evidence relating to K^+ efflux from contracting muscle is first reviewed; we then present the results of membrane potential measurements in mammalian muscles during maximal and submaximal contractions, and calculate the magnitude of the contribution to the resting potential by the electrogenic Na^+,K^+-pump. It will be shown that qualitative assessments of pump activity can be made in human muscles during voluntary or stimulated contractions, and also in the recovery period from fatigue. Finally, speculations are given as to the mechanisms responsible for increasing pump activity.

K^+ efflux during activity

[42]K has been used to measure K^+ efflux during impulse activity; in two early studies the mean value for single frog muscle fibres agreed closely with that for rat diaphragm, when

expressed per impulse and per cm^2 of membrane (9.6 pmole, Hodgkin & Huxley 1959a; 10.7 pmole, Creese et al. 1958). In the preparation used by Creese et al. (1958), some K$^+$ would have been carried back into the fibres by the Na$^+$,K$^+$-pump; hence the K$^+$ efflux in this and similar studies (see Sjøgaard 1990 for review) would have been underestimated, possibly by as much as 50% (Clausen & Everts 1988; see also Everts & Clausen 1988).

Experimental determinations of interstitial K$^+$ concentration.
The impulse-mediated increase in [K$^+$]$_e$, the interstitial K$^+$ concentration, can be measured directly, and also calculated from morphological and biochemical data. Neither approach is free from uncertainty, but both provide some indication of the changes that are likely to ensue during contraction. In the study by Hník et al. (1976) in the cat an ion-sensitive electrode was inserted into the femoral vein and all tributaries draining sources other than the gastrocnemius were ligated. The authors found that 50 Hz stimulation of this muscle raised [K$^+$]$_e$ from 4.8 mM to 8.2 mM, depending on the duration of the tetanus. Such values must be regarded as minimum estimates, however. Thus, the venous effluent will be a mixture of previously stagnant blood, which had accumulated K$^+$ during the tetanus, and of fresh inflow to the muscle. Also, there is no certainty that the interstitial fluid is in ionic equilibrium with the capillary plasma; the long time taken for [K$^+$] to return to normal values, at the end of a tetanus, suggests that diffusion of interstitial K$^+$ is impeded. The values of muscle [K$^+$]$_e$ in human subjects are likely to be further underestimated, because of the contamination of the muscle effluent with that from skin, subcutaneous tissue and non-contracting muscles; even so, mean values of 8.3 mM have been observed in femoral veins of subjects running on treadmills (Medbø & Sejersted 1990).

Measurements of [K$^+$]$_e$ in the muscle belly, made with ion-sensitive electrodes, might be expected to be more reliable. However, there are the possible effects of trauma, inflicted by the electrode, to consider; these might either increase [K$^+$]$_e$, by leakage of ions from damaged muscle fibres, or decrease it, by blocking impulses in those fibres round the electrode tip. Also spurious potentials, due to pressure at the electrode tip, may be comparable to those generated by changes in [K$^+$]. Finally, since the tips of the electrodes may be many times larger than the inter-fibre space (Hník et al. 1976; Juel 1986), their locations cannot be properly described as extracellular or intracellular. It is with these reservations in mind that such mean maximum values as 8.8 mM (Hník et al. 1976), and 10 mM (Juel 1986), must be considered.

The study by Vyskočil et al. (1983), though subject to the same sources of uncertainty, is particularly interesting since it was carried out in the intact human brachioradialis; the ion-sensitive electrode was introduced through a stainless steel trocar, before being advanced into the muscle tissue. Although the average [K$^+$]$_e$ rose from 4.5 mM to 9.5 mM, these authors showed a value of at least 15 mM being reached during a maximal contraction (see Fig. 2B of Vyskočil et al. 1983).

Theoretical determination of interstitial K$^+$ concentration.
The theoretical estimation of [K$^+$]$_e$ during a maximal voluntary contraction depends on surprisingly few assumptions. Thus, the K$^+$ efflux per impulse is known (see above), as are the dimensions of the muscle fibres and interstitial spaces and the motor unit firing rates during maximal voluntary contractions. Since the contraction is maximal, the intramuscular pressure will be well above that required to occlude the arterial inflow (Barcroft & Millen 1939; Sjøgaard 1990); hence the interstitial spaces and intramuscular capillaries can be considered as a closed compartment with diffusion of ions between one and the other. The

only major uncertainty is the extent of Na^+ and K^+ pumping between the interstitial spaces and the muscle fibres; in order to calculate the maximum possible rise in interstitial $[K^+]$, we shall ignore the effect of the pump.

Regarding fibre dimensions, an average value for the diameters of type I and type II fibres in the human biceps brachii muscle would be 50 μm (Brooke & Engel 1969), while transverse sections of the same muscle suggest that the inter-fibre distance is no more than 1 μm. If the fibres are considered as closely packed, 4-6 sided columns, then the interstitial space would be approximately 4% of the muscle volume, with the T-tubules adding a further 0.3% (Peachey 1965) and the capillaries 1-2%. A value of 6% for the extracellular space in skeletal muscles is much smaller than most biochemical estimates, for which chloride, inulin, and sucrose have been the most frequently used markers; it is likely that such estimates would be inflated by the connective tissue separating muscle fascicles and that surrounding the neurovascular bundles. More recently, however, Lindinger & Heigenhauser (1987) obtained mean values as low as 6.5% for some of the fast-twitch muscles in the rat, using mannitol as a marker. Taking these various considerations into account, it can be calculated by simple geometry that a single impulse will raise the interstitial $[K^+]$ by 0.2 mM.

How quickly will $[K^+]_e$ rise during a voluntary contraction? Firing rates greater than 100 Hz have been observed at the onset of maximal voluntary contractions of human hand muscles (Marsden et al. 1971), and a conservative value for the first few seconds of a muscle such as biceps brachii might be 25 Hz; such a value is obviously a global one, in the sense that some motor units have higher maximum firing rates than others (Freund et al. 1975). In a maximal contraction, all motor units will be recruited and, in one second, the interstitial $[K^+]$ could reach 5 mM (i.e. 25 x 0.2 mM). The amount of depolarization this rise might cause can be calculated from the following equation (Hodgkin 1958):

$$E_m = \frac{RT}{F} \log_e \frac{[K^+]_e + b\,[Na^+]_e}{[K^+]_i + b\,[Na^+]_i}$$

in which E_m is the membrane potential, and e and i denote extracellular and intracellular values; b is the ratio of the Na^+ and K^+ permeabilities of the muscle fibre membrane and is approximately 0.04 (see Hicks & McComas 1989). If allowances are made for changes in intracellular $[Na^+]$ and $[K^+]$ during contractile activity (see, for example, Sreter 1963), a rise of interstitial $[K^+]$ from 4 mM to 9 mM would depolarize a muscle fibre by approximately 14 mV, more than enough to cause impulse block.

On theoretical grounds, then, as little as one second of maximal effort would be expected to induce muscle paralysis. This surprising conclusion flies in the face of everyday experience, in which force can be maintained reasonably well for a minute or more; equally significant is the preservation of the muscle compound action potential (Bigland-Ritchie et al. 1982). Why are theory and observation so different? One reason is that the Cl⁻ conductance of the muscle fibre will tend to moderate the effects of a changing K^+ concentration gradient across the surface membrane, as reflected in the permeability and concentration terms for Cl⁻ in the Goldman-Hodgkin-Katz equation for membrane potential (cf. Goldman 1943). However, as shown by Hodgkin & Horowicz (1959b), the stabilizing effect of Cl⁻ is short-lived, due to redistribution of water and solute across the fibre membrane. Instead, it would appear that a second factor is more important in preventing K^+-induced paralysis; this factor is the electrogenic Na^+,K^+-pump.

Evidence for increased Na⁺,K⁺-pumping in muscle activity

Everts et al. (1988) showed, using ^{86}Rb, that there was a doubling of pump activity during stimulation of the isolated rat soleus at 2 Hz. The authors pointed out, however, that this increase was still far from the theoretical maximal rate of Na$^+$ and K$^+$ transport (cf. Clausen et al. 1987). A much earlier study, carried out on single frog semitendinosus muscle fibres, also showed a doubling of ^{24}Na extrusion during modest rates of stimulation (Hodgkin & Horowicz 1959a).

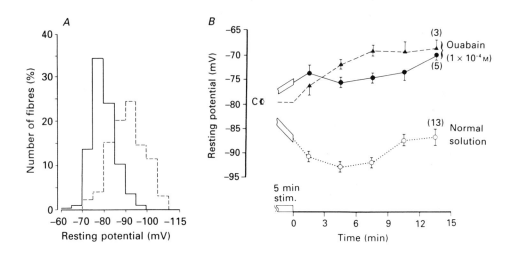

Figure 1,A. Effect of intermittent tetanic stimulation on rat muscle fibre membrane potentials; results in control and stimulated fibres shown by continuous and interrupted lines respectively. **B.** Abolition of tetanus-induced fibre hyperpolarization by ouabain (continuous line; stimulation period indicated by box). Other curves show effects of ouabain without stimulation (dashed line) and of stimulation without ouabain (dotted line). See text and Hicks & McComas 1989.

Physiological evidence for increased Na$^+$,K$^+$-pumping during muscle activity has been obtained in our own laboratory. In rat soleus muscles examined *in vivo*, Hicks & McComas (1989) observed that repeated tetani at 20 Hz increased the mean resting potential from -79.5 mV to -90.5 mV (Fig. 1,A). That this was due to the electrogenic effect of the Na$^+$,K$^+$-pump was shown by the absence of hyperpolarization if the experiments were repeated in the presence of ouabain or in the absence of extracellular K$^+$ (Fig. 1,B); cooling the muscle to 19°C produced a similarly negative result. Since the resting potentials of tetanized, but otherwise untreated, fibres were increased, the fibre action potentials enlarged by similar amounts and this, in turn, caused potentiation of the M-wave (muscle compound action potential). In surface fibres Hicks & McComas calculated that the Na$^+$,K$^+$-pump must be

The role of the Na$^+$, K$^+$-pump in delaying muscle fatigue contributing -20 mV to the resting potential; when stimulated fibres were challenged with 20 mM K^+ in the bathing fluid, the electrogenic component increased to -30 mV.

It is surprising that muscle fibre hyperpolarization had not been observed previously in investigations of muscle fatigue. The simplest explanation is that other workers have omitted protein in the bathing fluid, despite the earlier admonitions of Creese & Northover (1961) and Kernan (1963). As these last authors showed, the absence of protein leads to an increase in Na^+ permeability of the muscle fibre membrane *in vitro*, and to a depolarization of 10 mV or so.

Evidence for increased Na^+,K^+-pump activity in contracting human muscles.
There has long been evidence of augmented Na^+,K^+-pump activity during human muscle contractions in the phenomenon of 'pseudofacilitation', a term which describes the gradual increase in the amplitude of the M-wave during stimulated or voluntary activity. That the enlargement of the M-wave is not an artefact of tetanic stimulation, or of ischaemia, is demonstrated by similar findings during intermittent voluntary contractions of the intrinsic muscles of the hand, with the circulation intact (Hicks et al. 1989). In the past 'pseudofacilitation' has been attributed to greater synchronization of the individual muscle fibre action potentials, but there are good reasons for rejecting this explanation, certainly as a major cause (Hicks et al. 1989). Not infrequently, enlargement of the M-wave during stimulated or voluntary contraction has been recorded but without any comment as to its physiological significance or cellular mechanism; a recent example is the striking potentiation noted in single FF and F(int) motor units of the cat tibialis posterior muscle (Enoka et al. 1992).

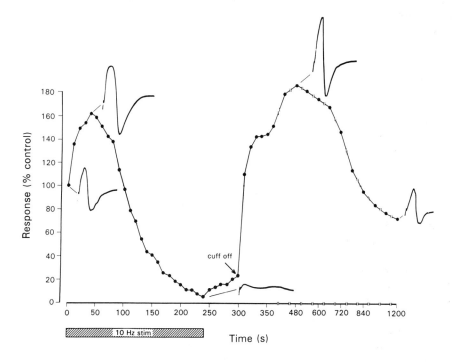

Figure 2. Changes in M-wave amplitude in biceps brachii muscle of a 20 yr old man, during 10 Hz stimulation, performed under ischaemic conditions; arterial cuff released at arrow (Galea, McComas & Einhorn, unpublished observations).

A.J. McComas, V. Galea, R.W. Einhorn, A.L. Hicks and S. Kuiack

On the basis of the animal studies, described above, it now seems certain that M-wave potentiation is largely due to the increased amplitudes of the muscle fibre action potentials, following pump-induced hyperpolarization. We have pursued M-wave studies in man, having discovered that the biceps brachii is a particularly favourable preparation for demonstrating facilitation (Fig. 2). By using arterial occlusion during this type of study, it has also been possible to document the time-course of recovery. It can be seen in Fig. 2 that the M-wave enlarges only slightly when tetanization is discontinued, provided ischaemia is maintained. As soon as the cuff is deflated, however, the M-wave amplitude rapidly increases; we attribute this change to the flushing out of K^+ from the interstitial spaces of the muscle, causing an instantaneous increase in the K^+ equilibrium potential, and hence in the muscle fibre resting potentials. There is then a slower potentiation which is maximal approximately three minutes after termination of ischaemia, and is probably due to increased Na^+,K^+-pumping (Galea & McComas 1991).

What happens during submaximal contractions?

Suppose only half the muscle fibres are contracting; what happens to the resting potentials of the other half? On *a priori* grounds, one might expect the inactive fibres to depolarize, due to the accumulation of K^+, released by the contracting fibres, in the interstitial fluid. To explore this possibility, Kuiack & McComas (1990, 1992) stimulated half of the ventral root axons innervating the rat soleus muscle and compared the resting potentials in the quiescent and previously-tetanized muscle fibres. They found that the quiescent fibres exhibited hyperpolarizations as large as those in the contracting fibres. This response is functionally advantageous, for it enables the quiescent fibres to be called into action as fatigue sets in, or if a stronger contraction is required.

Mechanism of increased Na^+,K^+-pump activity

It is probable that several mechanisms stimulate the Na^+,K^+-pump during muscle contraction. One factor will be the rise in *intracellular [Na^+]*, in keeping with the effects of direct stimulation of single muscle fibres (Hodgkin & Horowicz 1959a), and of Na^+ injection into neurones (Thomas 1972). However, in rat soleus muscles stimulated at 2 Hz, Everts et al. (1988) found a 63% increase in pumping, without any measurable increase in intracellular [Na^+]. The results of Kuiack & McComas (1990, 1992), using half-maximal contractions, also exclude intracellular Na^+ as the only factor stimulating the pump, since the non-tetanized fibres were also hyperpolarized. Similarly, a rise in interstitial [K^+] cannot be a major stimulus, since the effect of increasing [K^+]$_e$ in resting muscle is to *depolarize* the fibres (see, for example, Hicks & McComas 1989).

In contrast, there is evidence that *noradrenaline* may be a potent stimulus, since the contraction-induced hyperpolarization is abolished in the presence of propranolol, a ß-adrenergic blocker (Kuiack & McComas 1992; see, however, Everts et al. 1988). The source of noradrenaline in the muscle is presumably the sympathetic nerve fibres; in addition to those in the walls of the intramuscular arteries and arterioles (Fuxe & Sedvall 1965), there are others which end directly on the muscle fibres (Barker & Saito 1981) and might respond to action currents in the latter, as well as to efferent sympathetic drive. During voluntary contractions *adrenaline* may also stimulate the Na^+,K^+-pump but is clearly not essential, since M-wave enlargement in man is equally prominent in ischaemic as in non-ischaemic conditions (Galea & McComas 1991). Another possible pump stimulant is *CGRP* (calcitonin gene-related peptide) since this peptide is released from motor nerve endings (Uchida et al. 1990) and has recently been shown to enhance Na^+,K^+-transport in rat skeletal muscle (Clausen & Andersen 1991).

Summary of roles of the Na^+,K^+-pump in muscle contraction

In the paper we have concentrated on the electrogenic action of the Na^+,K^+-pump during muscle contraction. By contributing up to -30 mV to the resting membrane potentials, the pump is able to overcome the depolarizing tendency of the raised interstitial $[K^+]$ and to keep all the fibres in the muscle excitable. Further, the amount of pump activation appears to match the excitation frequency of the muscle fibres. Thus, even under ischaemic conditions, a full minute of non-decremental excitation of the fibres is guaranteed, at least, for frequencies up to 30 Hz (Galea & McComas, unpublished observations). The preservation of muscle fibre excitability is continued until force begins to decline, after which there is no longer any benefit in maintaining the resting membrane potential.

It is additionally possible that, by having a normal-sized or enlarged action potential at the surface membrane, effective excitation-contraction coupling is assured; thus, even if impulse conduction were to fail in the T-tubules, inward electrotonic spread of the surface signal might still be adequate to activate myofibrils in the centre of the fibre (Adrian et al. 1969).

The role of the Na^+,K^+-pump in restoring ionic equilibrium in the intracellular and extracellular compartments is equally important. Because of the limited pumping capacity, however, the exercise-induced changes in $[Na^+]$ and $[K^+]$ cannot be corrected as rapidly as the membrane potential; therefore the interstitial $[K^+]$ remains high at a time when the resting potential is normal or elevated.

Finally, by creating a membrane potential which is substantially above the K^+ equilibrium potential, the pump allows K^+ to diffuse passively down the transmembrane electrical gradient and into the fibre. It is to the advantage of the muscle fibre that the K^+ permeability should be high; it is possible that those K^+ channels which are opened by raised intracellular $[Ca^{2+}]$ (Pallotta et al. 1981) and by ATP deficiency (Spruce et al. 1987) have important roles in mediating the passive influx of K^+ during fatigue. This view is diametrically opposed to the one which proposes that such channels would further disrupt ionic homeostasis in fatigue, by promoting K^+ efflux (Sjøgaard 1990; Juel 1988).

Acknowledgments: We are indebted to MDAC, the Leman Brothers Muscular Dystrophy Foundation and NSERC for financial support. We are also grateful to Pat Holmes and Jane Butler for secretarial and editorial assistance.

References

Adrian RH, Costantin LL & Peachey LD (1969). Radial spread of contraction in frog muscle fibres. *Journal of Physiology* **204**, 231-257.

Barcroft H & Millen JLE (1939). The blood flow through muscle during sustained contraction. *Journal of Physiology* **97**, 17-31.

Barker D & Saito M (1981). Autonomic innervation of receptors and muscle fibres in cat skeletal muscle. *Proceedings of the Royal Society of London Series B* **212**,

317-332.

Bigland-Ritchie B, Kukulka CG, Lippold OCJ & Woods JJ (1982). The absence of neuromuscular transmission failure in sustained maximal voluntary contraction. *Journal of Physiology* **330**, 265-278.

Brooke MH & Engel WK (1969). The histographic analysis of human muscle biopsies with regard to fibre types. 1. Adult male and female. *Neurology* **19**, 221-233.

Clausen T & Andersen SV (1991). Calcitonin and calcitonin gene related peptide (CGRP) stimulate active Na,K-transport in rat skeletal muscle. *Acta Physiologica Scandinavica* **143**, 20A.

Clausen T & Everts ME (1991). K^+ induced inhibition of contractile force in rat skeletal muscle: role of active Na^+,K^+-transport. *American Journal of Physiology* **261**, C799-C807.

Clausen T & Everts ME (1988). Is the Na,K-pump capacity in skeletal muscle inadequate during sustained work? In: *Progress in Clinical and Biological Research*, **268**B, *The Na^+,K^+-pump*, Part B, Cellular aspects. Eds, Skou, JC et al. Alan Liss. New York. pp 239-244.

Clausen T, Everts ME & Kjeldsen K (1987). Quantification of the maximum capacity for active sodium-potassium transport in rat skeletal muscle. *Journal of Physiology* **388**, 163-181.

Creese R, Hashish SEE & Scholes NW (1958). Potassium movements in contracting diaphragm muscle. *Journal of Physiology* **143**, 307-324.

Creese R & Northover J (1961). Maintenance of isolated diaphragm with normal sodium content. *Journal of Physiology* **155**, 343-357.

Enoka RM, Trayanova N, Laouris Y, Bevan L, Reinking RM & Stuart DG (1992). Fatigue-related changes in motor unit action potentials of adult cats. *Muscle & Nerve* **14**, 138-150.

Everts ME & Clausen T (1988). Effects of thyroid hormone on Na^+-K^+ transport in resting and stimulated rat skeletal muscle. *American Journal of Physiology* **255**, E604-E612.

Everts ME, Retterstøl K & Clausen T (1988). Effects of adrenaline on excitation-induced stimulation of the sodium-potassium pump in rat skeletal muscle. *Acta Physiologica Scandinavica* **134**, 189-198.

Freund H-J, Buedingen H-J & Dietz V (1975). Activity of single motor units from forearm muscles during voluntary isometric contraction. *Journal of Neurophysiology* **38**, 933-946.

Fuxe K & Sedvall G (1965). The distribution of adrenergic nerve fibres to the blood vessels in skeletal muscle. *Acta Physiologica Scandinavica* **64**, 75-86.

Galea V & McComas AJ (1991). Effects of ischaemia on M-wave potentiation in human biceps brachii muscles. *Journal of Physiology* **438**, 212P.

Goldman DE (1943). Potential, impedance and rectification in membranes. *Journal of General Physiology* **27**, 37-60.

Hicks A, Fenton J, Garner S & McComas AJ (1989). M-wave potentiation during and after muscle activity. *Journal of Applied Physiology* **66**, 2606-2610.

Hicks A & McComas AJ (1989). Increased sodium pump activity following repetitive stimulation of rat soleus muscles. *Journal of Physiology* **414**, 337-349.

Hník P, Holas M, Krekule I, Křiž N, Majsnar J, Smieško V, Ujec E & Vyskočil F (1976). Work-induced potassium changes in skeletal muscle and effluent venous blood assessed by liquid ion-exchanger microelectrodes. *Pflügers Archiv* **362**, 85-94.

Hodgkin AL (1958). The Croonian Lecture: Ionic movements and electrical activity in giant nerve fibres. *Proceedings of the Royal Society of London Series B* **148**, 1-37.

Hodgkin AL & Horowicz P (1959a). Movements of Na and K in single muscle fibres. *Journal of Physiology* **145**, 405-432.

Hodgkin AL & Horowicz P (1959b). The influence of potassium and chloride ions in the membrane potential of single muscle fibres. *Journal of Physiology* **148**, 127-160.

Jones DA (1981). Muscle fatigue due to changes beyond the neuromuscular junction. In: *Human Muscle Fatigue: Physiological Mechanisms*. (CIBA Foundation Symposium, No. 82). Eds, Porter R & Whelan J. Pitman Medical. London. pp 178-192.

Juel C (1988). Is a Ca^{2+}-dependent K^+ channel involved in the K^+ loss from active muscles? *Acta Physiologica Scandinavica* **122**, P26.

Juel C (1986). Potassium and sodium shifts during in vitro isometric muscle contraction, and the time course of the ion-gradient recovery. *Pflügers Archiv* **406**, 458-463.

Kernan RP (1963). Resting potential of isolated rat muscles measured in plasma. *Nature (London)* **200**, 474-475.

Kuiack S & McComas AJ (1992). Transient hyperpolarization of non-contracting muscle fibres in anaesthetized rats. *Journal of Physiology. In press.*

Kuiack S & McComas AJ (1990). Transient hyperpolarization of non-contracting muscle fibres in anaesthetized rats. *Journal of Physiology* **426**, 29P.

Lindinger MI & Heigenhauser GJF (1987). Intracellular ion content of skeletal muscle measured by instrumental neutron activation analysis. *Journal of Applied Physiology* **63**, 426-433.

Marsden CD, Meadows JC & Merton P (1971). Isolated single motor units in human muscle and their rate of discharge during maximal voluntary effort. *Journal of Physiology* **217**, 12-13 P.

Medbø JI & Sejersted OM (1990). Plasma potassium changes with high intensity exercise. *Journal of Physiology* **421**, 105-122.

Pallotta BS, Magleby KL & Barrett JN (1981). Single channel recordings of Ca^{2+}-activated K^+ currents in rat muscle cell culture. *Nature (London)* **293**, 471-474.

Peachey LD (1965). The sarcoplasmic reticulum and transverse tubules of the frog's sartorius. *Journal of Cell Biology* **25**, 209-231.

Sjøgaard G (1990). Exercise-induced muscle fatigue: the significance of potassium. *Acta Physiologica Scandinavica* **140**, Suppl. 593, pp. 1-63.

Spruce AE, Standen NB & Stanfield PR (1987). Studies of the unitary properties of adenosine-5'-triphosphate-regulated channels of frog skeletal muscle. *Journal of Physiology* **382**, 213-236.

Sreter FA (1963). Distribution of water, sodium and potassium in resting and stimulated mammalian muscle. *Canadian Journal of Biochemistry and Physiology* **41**, 1035-1045.

Thomas RC (1972). Intracellular sodium activity and the sodium pump in snail neurons. *Journal of Physiology* **220**, 55-71.

Uchida S, Yamamoto H, Iio S, Matsumoto N, Wang X-B, Yonehara N, Imai Y, Inoki R & Yoshida H (1990). Release of calcitonin gene-related peptide-like immunoreactive substance from neuromuscular junction by nerve excitation and its action on striated muscle. *Journal of Neurochemistry* **54**, 1000-1003.

Vyskočil F, Hník P, Rehfeldt H, Vejspada R & Ujec E (1983). The measurements of K^+_e concentration changes in human muscles during volitional contractions. *Pflügers Archiv* **399**, 235-237.

Spectral compression of the EMG signal as an index of muscle fatigue

Carlo J. De Luca

NeuroMuscular Research Center and Dept. of Biomedical Engineering, Boston University, 44 Cummington St., Boston, MA 02215, USA

Abstract: Among Health Scientists, it has become customary for muscle fatigue to be described and evaluated in terms of the force that can be produced by a muscle. In the past decade this approach has been expanded to the assessment of voluntary contractions. Of particular concern is the use of the failure point of a muscle to produce a desired force as the event in time when the muscle becomes fatigued. This paper points out the limited usefulness and possible faulty interpretation of this approach. It is suggested that muscle fatigue is more correctly (and usefully) viewed as a continual function of contraction time. A technique that accomplishes this need is described and is referred to as the EMG spectral compression technique. This technique is based on the well-known fact that the frequency spectrum of the EMG signal is continuously compressed during a sustained contraction. The median frequency of the EMG signal is recommended as the preferred variable for tracking spectral compression. It is shown that the median frequency is affected mostly by the pH in the muscle, which depends on the amount of net Lactate that is produced and removed, as well as some other unknown factor(s). It is argued that this objective and non-invasive, non-painful technique provides superior means for assessing and monitoring muscle fatigue in humans performing voluntary contractions. It also provides convenient means for studying some biochemical modifications within the muscle without invading the muscle.

Muscle performance

Muscles are physiological force actuators. Thus, among those trained in the Health Sciences it has been teleologically reasonable to evaluate the performance of muscles by the behavior of the force that they generate. Therefore, it is not surprising that early attempts at measuring the deterioration in the capability to maintain a desired performance level (muscle fatigue) would be based on a decrease in the force output of the muscle.

Pursuing this line of thought, Burke *et al.* (1971) described a fatigue test for classifying the performance of muscle fibers which could be stimulated directly via an electrical pulse train (40 Hz; 1/3 s on, 2/3 s off) applied to the nerve innervating the muscle. The performance of the muscle fiber was assessed by observing the amplitude of the force twitch. When the amplitude began to decrease, fatigue was considered to begin. This approach made reasonable use of the force variable as an index of muscle fatigue, but introduced a notion of fatigue that was related to an indication of a deterministic failure in the behavior of the monitored variable. This approach has been widely accepted and as a consequence, the notion of fatigue has become synonymous with the concept of failure as used in engineering and physics, two disciplines that have dealt with the concept of fatigue for considerable time. Following the lead of Burke, Edwards (1981) extended this concept of fatigue to voluntary contractions in the human by describing fatigue as the inability to sustain a voluntary contraction at a predetermined force level. More recently, Bigland-Ritchie (1984) has advanced the concept of monitoring the rate of decline of force output during a sustained maximal voluntary contraction. Although this approach improves on the use of force as the variable of measure, it remains susceptible to the capability and/or willingness of the individual to continue to elicit maximal effort during a test. Such tests are uncomfortable and questionably objective.

The notion of *equating fatigue to a failure point* carries with it some practical disadvantages. For example, fatigue would be detectable only after it has occurred. This approach would have little use in clinical and ergonomics applications where it is often desirable to have indications that precede failure to produce the desired force so that appropriate remedies can be made or evaluations can be taken. Conceptually, the notion of the failure point also relates to the occurrence of a catastrophic event. During a sustained contraction, a complex system which has numerous individual processes simultaneously operating to achieve an end goal is at work. Consider for example the metabolite usage, the Lactate accumulation (with its corresponding pH changes), modifications in the Calcium ion release mechanism, Potassium ion losses, Creatine Phosphate usage, decrease in the firing rates, motor force-twitch potentiation and other mechanisms. All of these processes undergo continual modification as a function of time during a contraction. Each process fatigues at its own rate and most, if not all, affect the ability of the muscle to produce force. Thus, failure to produce force may occur either by a catastrophic event in a dominant process or as a combination of the fatigue characteristics of the individual processes.

The use of force during a voluntary contraction as an index of muscle fatigue introduces at least three additional confounding factors. Firstly, in voluntary contractions the force output of an individual muscle is not often directly accessible. Without surgical intervention, one can only measure the net torque at a joint. That is, the difference between the torques produced by the agonist muscles and the torque produced by the antagonist muscles. Thus, the monitored torque may not faithfully represent the torque (or force) of the muscle of interest, depending on the behavior of the antagonist muscles. This issue is particularly troublesome in the presence of pain or injury where muscles may alter their load sharing during a task. Secondly, during a submaximal contraction, it is possible to maintain the torque (or force) output acceptably constant in a macroscopic sense, but there are time-dependent physiological and biochemical processes that microscopically alter the means for generating force during a sustained contraction. Some of these are: 1) some motor units might become derecruited, 2) the force twitches of motor units potentiate, i. e., the integral of their force increases, and 3) the firing rates of most active motor units decrease. This later phenomenon was first reported by Person and Kudina (1972) and independently by De Luca and Forrest (1973). Later, De Luca (1979) proposed " ... if the firing rate of the motor unit decreases and there is no significant recruitment, a complimentary mechanism must occur to maintain the constant-force output. One possible mechanism is the potentiation of force twitch tension of the motor units as a contraction progresses." An additional caveat was added by De Luca et al. (1982a) "...that this behavior is likely to be due either to post-tetanic twitch potentiation or to a concurrent reduction in the force output of agonist and antagonist muscles which maintains the monitored force output of a joint constant". Now this concept has been adopted into the motor control literature. Thirdly, during a voluntary contraction the failure point is a function of both physiological and psychological factors, and it is difficult to know accurately the causal relationship of each to the failure point.

The psychological factor could be removed by activating the muscle via electrical stimulation instead of a voluntary effort. However, a muscle contraction induced by electrical activation generates force by decidedly different means. For a review of electrical stimulation of muscles see Merletti, Knaflitz and De Luca (1992). By contemporary methodologies, the electrical stimulation is delivered as a train of pulses at a fixed frequency, usually 30-40 Hz, whereas in actuality the firing rates of the motor units are quasi-random. Also, the recruitment order of the motor units is decidedly different than in the natural activation. Although the order is not completely reversed, whether the motor point of the muscle is stimulated (Knaflitz, Merletti and De Luca: 1990) or the nerve is stimulated (Gorman & Mortimer, 1983, among others). But most importantly during electrical stimulation, the higher threshold motor units, which decrease their force output more quickly than others, are stimulated at a much higher rate than occurs during natural activation. During a voluntary contraction, the higher threshold motor units fire at lower rates than earlier recruited, lower threshold motor units (De Luca et al., 1982b). *The central nervous system appears to be designed to compromise between activating the muscle to generate the maximal force possible and sustaining a contraction for a finite amount of time.*

If not force, then what?

The other obvious variable that has been commonly used to assess the performance of muscles is the surface electromyographic (EMG) signal. This approach presents several advantages: 1) The EMG signal can be detected from a specific muscle designated for study, unlike the force variable which cannot be easily isolated for an individual muscle. However, if it is desired to study a group of muscles, multiple channel detection techniques may be used to obtain the required EMG signals simultaneously. 2) The EMG signal provides information that directly and objectively relates to the state of the muscle studied; it reflects the factors that are directly related to the anatomy or architecture, the physiology and the biochemistry of the muscle. 3) It circumvents the subjectivity of the voluntary-force variable monitored during a voluntary contraction. 4) Detection techniques are not painful and are not invasive, rendering them useful for clinical and ergonomics purposes.

Early attempts at using the EMG signal as an index of muscle fatigue relied on the amplitude of the signal, with inconsistent success. It has been known for over four decades (Knowlton *et al.*, 1951) that the amplitude of the EMG signal generally increases during sustained sub-maximal constant-force contractions. This phenomenon is due to the increased time duration of the motor unit action potentials (MUAP) during a sustained contraction. It will be seen below that this behavior is more reliably and clearly displayed in the behavior of the frequency spectrum of the EMG signal. Also, amplitude measurements of the EMG signal are prone to be affected by various sources of noise and impedance matching complications. The electrical noise can originate from the ambient surroundings, improper grounding of the electronic equipment, low-quality amplifiers, electrically-unstable connection to the skin by the electrodes caused by ineffective mechanical coupling of the electrode to the skin, movement of the electrode with respect to the skin causing motion artifacts, and other more esoteric sources.

An alternative and more reliable approach is to study the behavior of the EMG signal in the frequency domain. This is known as the EMG spectral technique. Modifications in the EMG signal during a sustained contraction which are difficult to quantify in the time domain can become considerably easier to quantify in the frequency domain. However, this technique is not without its own set of complications; they will be discussed in a section near the end of the paper.

The EMG spectral variable technique

It is well known that during a sustained contraction the surface EMG signal undergoes a translation (slowing) in the time domain. This phenomenon can be seen in the top right-hand quadrant of Figure 1, where examples of the EMG signal detected at the beginning and end of an isometric constant-force contraction are shown. If the Fourier transforms of the two signals are taken, the slowing of the EMG signal is seen as a compression in the frequency domain. That is, the amplitude of the low-frequency components increases and that of the high-frequency components decreases. (To be precise, the spectrum also undergoes a mild change in shape that is not explainable by a compression in the frequency domain. See Brody *et al.* (1991) and Merletti, Knaflitz and De Luca (1992).) A convenient means of tracking the frequency compression is to monitor the median frequency of the spectrum. For an overview see Figure 1 and for details see a review article by De Luca (1985).

The cause of the frequency compression provides reason for using the spectral technique as an index of muscle fatigue. Through mathematical modeling and experimentation we have established that the control properties of the motor units (firing rate and synchronization) do not affect the frequency spectrum appreciably (De Luca 1985). The now well known decrease in the firing rates of the motor unit during constant force contractions cause only a minor shift in the frequency spectrum below 40 Hz.

Synchronization among the discharges of concurrently active motor units has been, at times, used to explain the modification in the frequency spectrum. Recent work at our Center has indicated that only approximately 4-5 % of motor unit discharges are synchronized, and that these discharges occur in bursts of mostly one or two consecutive firings at sporadic intervals throughout the contraction. These observations strongly suggest that synchronization cannot be an influential factor in modifying the frequency spectrum.

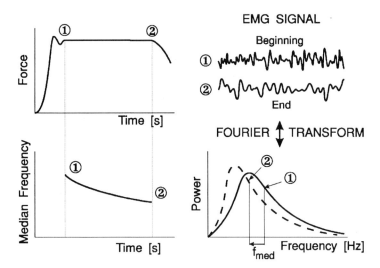

Figure 1. The EMG signal at the beginning (1) and the end (2) of a constant-force isometric contraction (top left quadrant), along with the corresponding frequency spectral compression and the time course of the median frequency during the sustained contraction. This is a schematic representation consistent with the behavior of the real data.

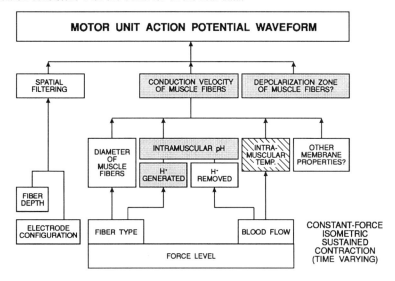

Figure 2. Factors which effect the shape of the motor unit action potential during a sustained contraction. The shaded boxes indicate factors that modify as function of time during a sustained constant-force isometric contraction above 30 % MVC. Temperature is less relevant than the other highlighted factors. Other indicated factors are relevant only during weaker contractions or non-isometric contractions.

The explanation for the frequency compression can be found in the behavior of the MUAP shape during a contraction. This is the likely source because we know from mathematical modeling that the shape of the frequency spectrum of the EMG signal is almost exclusively due to the shape of the constituent MUAPs. For the past decade my colleagues (notably Serge Roy and Roberto Merletti) have been attempting to understand which factors dominate the behavior of MUAP shape. Our current understanding is summarized in Figure 2, which presents the known influences on the MUAP shape, and highlights those that are subject to modification during a sustained constant-force contraction. These influences progressively affect the MUAP shape during the accumulation of fatigue. The two dominant factors are the conduction velocity (CV) of the muscle fibers and some other, yet to be identified factor. We suspect the length of the depolarization zone to be that other factor (Merletti, Knaflitz, De Luca; 1992), but Stegeman (in this book) suspects otherwise.

The modeling work of Lindstrom et al. (1970) as well as our own modeling work (Stulen & De Luca, 1981) has shown that the CV of the muscle fibers directly affects the bandwidth of the frequency spectrum and inversely (by a square-root factor) the amplitude of the EMG signal. In the past decade there have been several reports from different laboratories which agree that the CV of muscles fibers decreases during a sustained contraction. Teleologically, the causal relationship between CV and EMG spectral compression can be seen in Figure 3. In this figure, the depolarization zone of a muscle fiber is seen moving past a pair of (differential) electrodes. The slower the CV, the longer will be the time taken by the depolarization zone to pass by the electrodes, and consequently the duration of the detected action potential will be longer. An increased duration of the action potential is reminiscent of the "slowing down" of the EMG signal mentioned at the beginning of this section and causes its frequency spectrum to compress. It should be noted that the arguable effect of the increased depolarization zone can be explained in a similar fashion. That is, if the depolarization zone increases during a sustained contraction, it will take more time for it to pass by the detection electrodes and the time duration of the action potential will increase correspondingly.

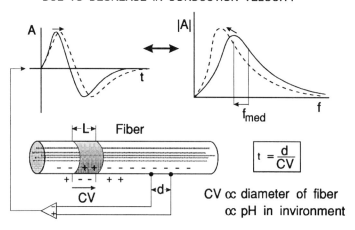

Figure 3. A schematic representation of the causal relationship between the conduction velocity along the muscle fibers and the time duration and spectrum of the detected action potential.

Now the question remains as to what causes the CV to decrease. Recent work in our Center (Brody et al.; 1991) demonstrated that the pH of the fluid surrounding the muscle fibers has a profound and causal effect on the CV. In this study, we placed a rat diaphragm nerve-muscle preparation in a bath of Ringer solution into which CO_2, O_2 and N_2 could be aerated to change the pH of the solution. The pH was fixed at 6.6, 7.0 and 7.4. At each pH setting, the nerve was stimulated supramaximally for 3 s with a pulse train of 40 Hz. The EMG signal from the muscle was detected by a three-bar electrode and amplified with a double-differential configuration. This method enabled us to separately and simultaneously measure the median frequency and the CV from the same set of EMG signals. In this fashion we found that at the beginning of a contraction (in the first 0.1 s, prior to any significant fatigue) the CV was directly related to the pH value. That is, when the pH was decreased, the time duration of the compound action potential increased and the amplitude decreased; the opposite occurred when the pH was increased. But, the change in the time duration and amplitude were completely accounted for by the corresponding change in the CV. See Figure 4a which compares the compound action potential shapes with the amplitude normalized by the inverse of the CV and the time duration by the CV at each pH level. However, at the end of the sustained 3 s stimulation, the change in the time duration and amplitude of the compound action potential could not be completely accounted for by the change in the CV at the different time intervals; indicating that some other(s) causative agent affected the shape of the compound action potential. See Figure 4b. In particular, the later part of the compound action potential could not be matched, indicating that the recovery phase is slowed down as a function of contraction time. One possible cause for this effect might be the leakage of Potassium ions from the membrane, however, this suggestion remains to be proven.

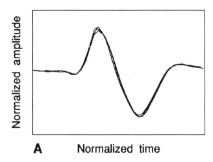 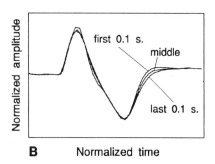

Figure 4A. The shape of the compound action potential detected from the stimulated rat diaphragm muscle at pH = 6.6, 7.0, 7.4. The amplitude and the time scales have been normalized by the conduction velocity value at the corresponding pH. Note the similarity of the shapes. (See text for explanation.)

Figure 4B. The shape of the compound action potential at a set pH at the beginning (0 - 0.1 s), middle and end (2.9 - 3.0 s) of a stimulated contraction. The amplitude and time scales are normalized by the conduction velocity values at the corresponding times. Note that the normalized shapes are not identical. (See text for explanation.)

The amount of pH change is a function of the Lactate that is generated and removed from the muscle fiber environment. Work in progress in our Center indicates that, as anticipated, the fiber type influences the change in the median frequency, with greater changes seen in muscles which contain large proportions of anaerobic Type II fibers (Extensor Digitorum Longus) than those rich in Type I fibers (Soleus) of the rat. This observation was suspected in our earlier work (Merletti, Sabbahi & De Luca; 1984) where the median frequency was measured in the human First Dorsal Interosseous before, during and after ischemia was induced in constant-force isometric contractions at 20 % and 80 % of maximal voluntary contraction (MVC). In that study, the decrease in the median frequency during the contractions was dramatically higher in the 80 % MVC, where the Type II fibers are activated in considerably greater quantity. Thus, the force level of a contraction is critically important when using the EMG spectral technique for at least three reasons:

1) Larger diameter fibers (recruited in greater proportion at higher force levels) have larger CVs which produce MUAPs of shorter time duration and higher frequency bandwidths. This yields higher initial values of the median frequency at the beginning of a contraction. See Broman, Bilotto & De Luca (1985).

2) Anaerobic Type II fibers (recruited in greater proportion at higher force levels) increase the rate

of Lactate production and decreases the pH during a contraction. This yields higher rate of decrease for the median frequency during a contraction.

3) Blood flow (which is shut off at higher force levels) determines the amount of Lactate that remains in the environment of the muscle fibers. This affects the value of the median frequency. At force levels above 30 % MVC, in most muscles, the blood flow is occluded.

In addition to the concern over the force level, it is also important to monitor the length changes in the muscle during a contraction. Because the electrode is fixed on the skin above the muscle, any change in the muscle length will change the relative distance between the electrode and the active fibers. This would modify the spatial filtering characteristics and thus affect the shape of the MUAP with a corresponding effect on the median frequency.

It is recommended that the EMG spectral technique be used during constant-force isometric contractions above 30 % MVC. If it is to be applied to dynamic contractions, then the median frequency should be compared only when the EMG signal is reasonably stationary and detected at the same phase during a repetitive dynamic contraction. If the values of the median frequency are to be compared across individuals, then the amount of fatty tissue beneath the skin becomes a factor of concern because it affects the spatial filtering characteristics.

Proper use of a new technique:

When a new technique is used in the research and clinical environments, it is incumbent on the users to apply it with proper respect for and knowledge of its limitations and idiosyncrasies. All new technology has unexplored fringes that require careful considerations. Unchecked usage will provide inconsistent and possibly conflicting results. When using the EMG spectral technique the following technical considerations must be respected:

1) The electrode should be sufficiently small and placed well within the borders of the muscle so as to detect the EMG signal from the muscle in question and not crosstalk signal from adjacent muscles. Signals from adjacent muscles will be subjected to greater spatial filtering, thus reducing the value of the spectral variables of the detected signals. We have developed a special electrode, which in most cases, can satisfy the two conditions. The detection surfaces of our electrode consist of two parallel bars, each 1.0 cm long and 1.0 mm wide spaced 1.0 cm apart.

2) The spacing between the detection surfaces inversely scales the value of the spectral variables.

3) The orientation of the detection surfaces with respect to the muscle fibers also affects the value of the spectral variables.

4) The temperature of the muscle directly affects the spectral variables. Tests made for comparison should be made at similar temperatures or scaled appropriately.

5) Ambient electromagnetic radiation, motion artifacts, clipping of the signal during detection, and poor signal-to-noise ratio all adversely affect the value of the EMG spectral variables.

Final note

Given that both the EMG spectral variables and the force variable of the contractile mechanisms undergo changes during the progression of fatigue, it is inevitable to ask if a relationship exists between the two. The answer is undoubtedly yes. The more interesting question is if the relationship is causal. This issue is not clear at this time, and a considerable amount of work is required before meaningful statements can be made to illuminate this issue. Nonetheless the lack of proof of a causal relationship does not logically preclude the use of the spectral variables as a fatigue index, especially when empirical evidence reveals its usefulness. For example, work in progress at our Center (Roy , De Luca & Casavant, 1989) as well as corroborative work by others (Biederman et al., in press) this technique has been successfully adapted to objectively assess muscle impairment associated with lower back pain disorders. Results have demonstrated characteristic "patterns" of EMG median frequency that are reliably different for individuals with muscle insufficiency associated with lower back pain.

Acknowledgements: The author wishes to thank all his colleagues and students, who over the years have contributed, in different ways, to the work described in this paper; among them Drs. Serge Roy and Roberto Merletti are noteworthy. This work was supported by Liberty Mutual Insurance Company and the Rehabilitation Research and Development Service of the Department of Veterans Affairs.

References

Biedermann HJ, Shanks GL, Forrest WJ & Inglis J (In Press). Power spectrum analyses of electromyographic activity: discriminators in the differential assessment of patients with chronic low back pain. *Spine.*

Bigland-Ritchie B & Woods JJ. (1984) Changes in muscle contractile properties and neural control during human muscular fatigue. *Muscle and Nerve* **7**, 691-699.

Brody LR, Pollock MT, Roy SH, De Luca CJ & Celli B (1991). pH-induced effects on media n frequency and conduction velocity of the myoelectric signal. *Journal of Applied Physiology* **71**, 1878-1885.

Broman H, Bilotto G & De Luca CJ (1985). Myoelectric signal conduction velocity and spectral parameters: Influence of force and time. *Journal of Applied Physiology* **58**, 1428-1437.

Burke R E, Levine D N, Zajac III F E, Tsairis P & Engel W K (1971). Mammalian motor units: Physiological-histochemical correlation in three types in cat gastrocnemius. *Science* **174**, 709-712.

De Luca CJ & Forrest WJ (1973). Some properties of motor unit action potential trains recorded during constant force isometric contractions in man. *Kybernetik* **12**, 160-168.

De Luca CJ (1979). Physiology and Mathematics of Myoelectric Signals. *IEEE Transactions on Biomedical Engineering* **26**, 313-325.

De Luca CJ (1985). Myoelectric manifestations of localized muscular fatigue. *CRC Critical Reviews in Biomedical Engineering* **11**, 251-279.

De Luca CJ, LeFever RS, McCue MP & Xenakis AP (1982a) Control scheme governing concurrently active human motor units during voluntary contractions. *Journal of Physiology* **329**, 129-142.

De Luca CJ, LeFever RS, McCue MP & Xenakis AP (1982b). Behaviour of human motor units in different muscles during linearly-varying contractions. *Journal of Physiology* **329**, 113-128.

Edwards RHT (1981) Human muscle function and fatigue. In: *Human Muscle Fatigue: Physiological Mechanisms.* (Ciba Foundation Symposium No.82) Eds Porter R and Whelan J. Pitman Medical. London. 1-18.

Gorman P H & Mortimer JT (1983). The effect of stimulus parameters on the recruitment characteristics of direct nerve stimulation. *IEEE Transactions BME* **30**, 407.

Knaflitz M, Merletti R, & De Luca CJ (1990). Inference of motor unit recruitment order in voluntary and electrically elicited contractions. *Journal of Applied Physiology* **68**, 1657- 1667.

Knowlton GC, Bennett RL & McClure R (1951). Electromyography of fatigue. *Archives of Physical Medicine* **32**, 648.

Lindstrom L, Magnusson R & Petersen I (1970). Muscular fatigue and action potential conduction velocity changes studied with frequency analysis of EMG signals. *Electromyography* **10**, 341.

Merletti R, Knaflitz M & De Luca CJ (1992). Electrically Evoked Myoelectric Signals. *Critical Reviews in Biomedical Engineering* **19**, 293-340.

Merletti R, Sabbahi MA & De Luca CJ (1984). Median frequency of the myoelectric signal: Effects of ischemia and cooling. *European Journal of Applied Physiology* **52**, 258-265.

Person RS & Kudina LP (1972). Discharge frequency and discharge pattern in human motor units during voluntary contractions of muscle. *EEG and Clinical Neurophysiology*, 471-483.

Roy SH, De Luca CJ & Casavant DA (1989). Lumbar muscle fatigue and chronic low back pain. *Spine* **14**, 992-1001.

Stulen FB & De Luca CJ (1981). Frequency parameters of the myoelectric signal as a measure of muscle conduction velocity. *IEEE Transaction Biomedical Engineering* **28**, 515.

Changes of intracellular fibre action potentials and the surface EMG: a simulation study of fatigue

D.F. Stegeman, W.H.J.P. Linssen

Research Group on Neuromuscular Disorders, Dept. of Neurology,
University of Nijmegen, P.O. Box 9101, 6500 HB Nijmegen, The Netherlands

Intracellular muscle fibre action potentials (IAPs) are influenced by local muscular fatigue (Hanson & Persson 1971, Lännergren & Westerblad 1987). It is known that surface EMG (SEMG) characteristics are largely dependent on these electrophysiological changes at the sarcolemma (Lateva 1988). The study presented here aimed at a transparent, model-based, quantification of the influence of changes at the single fibre level on major SEMG characteristics (*RMS* amplitude and median frequency *Fmed*).

Methods of calculation

The IAP is characterized by three parameters, mean amplitude *A*, mean duration *T* and mean fibre conduction velocity (MFCV) *U* . The calculation of extracellular single fibre action potentials (SFAPs) uses volume conduction theory. A motor unit action potential (MUAP) is modelled as the sum of bipolarly recorded SFAPs, dispersed in arrival time at the electrode (Lindström & Magnusson 1977). The dispersion is caused by fibre size differences and lengths of end-plate regions within a motor unit. The finiteness of the muscle fibres and of the volume conductor (Gootzen et al. 1991) can be omitted within the present scope. In the presented results it is assumed that the central motor drive has fixed properties. So, all simulated changes in *Fmed* and *RMS* are exclusively caused by changing fibre membrane properties (see for more details Stegeman & Linssen 1992).

Results

Results can be expressed in three statements on *RMS* and *Fmed*:
(1) Volume conductor differences, e.g. the distance between a motor unit and the electrode and the (electrical) conductivities of the tissue, dominate the absolute values

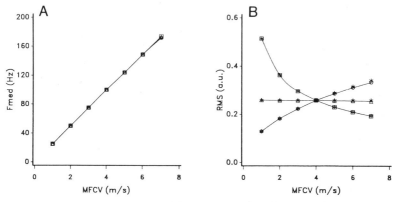

Figure 1 A-B. Predicted influence of MFCV on *Fmed* (part A) and *RMS* (part B). Various symbols point to different assumptions with respect to the not quantitatively known dependence of the IAP duration *T* in relation to MFCV (*U*). **Squares**: $T=4/U$ ms (constant spatial length of IAP), **circles**: $T=1$ ms (constant duration of IAP), **triangles**: $T=(4/U)^{\frac{1}{2}}$ (intermediate assumption). Asterisks in part B show the behaviour of the equation at point (2) in the results section.

of *Fmed* and *RMS*. Volume conduction does not interfere, however, with the relative (percentual) fatigue induced changes in *Fmed* and *RMS* as far as they are the result of IAP changes (not shown).

(2) *RMS* is almost proportionally dependent on the spatial extension *L* of the IAP (*L=T U*) and on *A*. It is inversely proportional to the square root of MFCV ($U^{-½}$).
In combination: $$RMS = C_1 \, A \, T \, U^{½}$$ (see Fig.1B asterisks).

(3) *Fmed* is about proportionally dependent on *U*, independent of *A*, and almost independent of *T*: $$Fmed = C_2 \, U$$ (see Fig.1A).

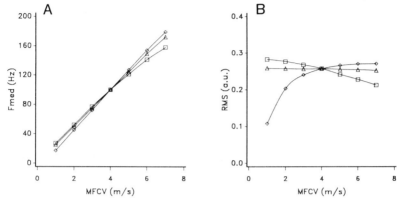

Figure 2 A-B. Results of different assumptions with respect to SFAP temporal dispersion changes with *U* within a motor unit **(triangles**: as in Fig. 1, dispersion scaled with U^{-1} (no fatiguability difference between fibres); **squares**: no dependence of the dispersion on *U* (higher fatigue resistance of thinner fibres); **diamonds**: dispersion scaled with U^{-2} (higher fatigue resistance of thicker fibres).

Discussion

The influence of IAP characteristics on SEMG changes can be described by the above simple relations quite accurately (Fig. 1). An assumption for these relations to be valid is that a motor unit must be homogeneous with respect to the fatigue resistance of its constituent fibres (Fig. 2). Quantitative basic experimental knowledge on the relation between *U*, which can be measured under *in situ* conditions, and the more difficult to obtain other IAP parameters (*A*, *T*) is scarce. This knowledge would, together with models as presented, support interpretation of SEMG parameters under fatiguing circumstances. To put it more strongly, in particular SEMG amplitude changes can hardly be interpreted without such knowledge.

References

Gootzen THJM, Stegeman DF, Van Oosterom A (1991). Finite limb dimensions and finite muscle length in a model for the generation of electromyographic signals. *Electroencephalography and Clinical Neurophysiology* 81:152-162.

Hanson J, Persson A (1971). Changes in the action potential and contraction of isolated frog muscle after repetitive stimulation. *Acta Physiologica Scandinavia* 81:340-348.

Lännergren J, Westerblad H (1987). Action potential fatigue in single skeletal muscle fibres of Xenopus. *Acta Physiologica Scandinavia* 129:311-318.

Lateva ZC (1988). Dependence of quantitative parameters of the extracellular potential power spectrum on propagation velocity, duration and asymmetry of action potentials. *Electromyography and Clinical Neurophysiology* 28:191-203.

Lindström LH, Magnusson RI (1977). Interpretation of myoelectric power spectra: a model and its applications. *Proceedings of the IEEE* 65:653-662.

Stegeman DF, Linssen WHJP (1992). Muscle fibre action potential changes and surface EMG: a simulation study. *Journal of Electromyography and Kinesiology* (submitted).

Intrinsic hand muscles: unexpected differences in fatigue-associated EMG-behaviour

C. Zijdewind and D. Kernell

Department of Neurophysiology, Academisch Medisch Centrum, University of Amsterdam, Meibergdreef 15, 1105 AZ Amsterdam, The Netherlands

Introduction

Small muscles of the human hand are often used for the study of neuromuscular fatigue. We have been investigating the fatigue-associated electromyographic (EMG) behaviour of two frequently used muscles: the *adductor pollicis* (AP; adductor of the thumb) and the *first dorsal interosseus* (FDI; abductor of the index finger). These muscles are known to differ in their histochemical fibre-type composition; AP has about 80% type I fibres, whereas FDI has a more evenly balanced composition (57% type I fibres, Johnson et al. 1973). Therefore one might expect a difference in fatigue-associated EMG behaviour between AP and FDI.

Methods

The results were obtained from the right hand of 16 healthy right-handed volunteers (8 male, 8 female). The hand and forearm of the subjects were immobilized with pressure plates and velcro tape, while the index finger was positioned at an angle of about 80% of maximal abduction. Transcutaneous electrical stimulation was given to the ulnar nerve (0.1 ms pulses, 50% supramaximal intensity). The fatigue test consisted of bursts (30 Hz; 10 pulses) repeated once a second during 5 minutes. During the fatigue test force recordings were made for thumb (adduction) and index-finger (abduction/adduction, flexion). Monopolar EMG recording electrodes were attached to the skin overlying the AP and the FDI belly. Measurements of EMG reactions during fatigue tests concerned peak-to-peak amplitude and half-area (area of the first negative peak) of compound action potentials (M-waves), as analyzed for the first and tenth M-wave of each burst.

TABLE 1. Fatigue-associated EMG-behaviour in AP and FDI, as measured for the first M-wave of each burst in different groups of subjects.
*All values are expressed as ratios (%) of measurements obtained at the end of a fatigue test vs. those for the initial burst. Significance of differences for AP vs. FDI (paired t test) and for male vs. female (t test) indicated by: ** for $P < 0.01$, * for $P < 0.05$, ns for not significant, i.e. $P > 0.05$).*

| | --- M-wave amplitude --- | | | --- M-wave half-area --- | | |
	AP	AP vs FDI	FDI	AP	AP vs FDI	FDI
All subjects	94	ns	90	97	ns	90
Male (M)	107	**	89	110	*	99
Female (F)	81	*	90	82	ns	81
M vs F	**		ns	**		ns

Results

When analyzing the EMG recordings for all subjects together, no significant differences were found between FDI and AP (Table 1). However, when considering the results for male and female subjects separately, significant differences became apparent:

1) between AP and FDI of the same individuals (Table 1), and

2) between males and females for the same muscles, this was valid for FDI initially (Fig. 1) and for AP later on during the test (Table 1, Fig.1).

When analyzed at corresponding times within the fatigue tests, no significant differences were found between males and females with respect to the fatigue-associated drop in the force of thumb adduction (AP contraction). Forces of the index finger, as caused by electrical ulnar-nerve stimulation, are of complex origin and will be dealt with elsewhere (Zijdewind and Kernell, in preparation).

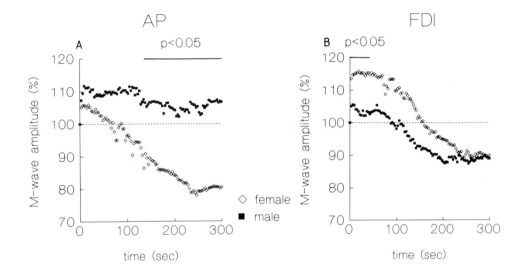

Figure 1. Relative changes in M-wave amplitude (% of initial value; first M-wave per burst) during simultaneous fatigue tests of AP and FDI. Means plotted for males (n=8) and females (n=8). Times during which values of males and females were significantly different from each other indicated by bars (paired t tests, P<0.05).

Discussion

In accordance with our general expectations, differences were indeed found between the fatigue-associated EMG reactions of AP and FDI. The observed differences between males and females were, however, completely unexpected. Further studies will be necessary for establishing whether these differences were caused by truly sex-linked variations in muscle characteristics or whether other sex-associated factors were of influence on the EMG recordings (e.g. possible effects on recording situation of differences in hand size, possible differences in local temperature control, etc.).

Reference

Johnson MA, Polgar J, Weightman D & Appleton D (1973). Data on the distribution of fibre types in thirty-six human muscles. An autopsy study. *Journal of the Neurological Sciences* **18**, 111-129.

C. Zijdewind and D. Kernell

Reaction of end-plate potentials in slow and fast rat muscle during fatigue-test stimulation

O. Eerbeek and D. Kernell

Department of Neurophysiology, Academisch Medisch Centrum, University of Amsterdam, Meibergdreef 15, 1105 AZ Amsterdam, The Netherlands.

It is well known that, during electrically induced fatigue tests, a decline in force ('force fatigue') is commonly associated with a decrease in amplitude of the evoked compound action potentials ('EMG depression'). In rats, the slowly contracting soleus muscle (Sol) is more resistant to both force fatigue and EMG depression than the fast extensor digitorum longus muscle (EDL) (e.g. Enoka et al. 1989; cf. Figs.1A, 2A). As part of our efforts to elucidate the possible causes for these differences in EMG-depression, we have now compared the two muscles with regard to the fatigue-test associated behaviour of their end-plate potentials (EPPs).

Nerve-muscle preparations from normal adult rats (250-300 g body weight) were mounted in an in vitro chamber, which was perfused at a rate of 30-40 ml/min with Krebs solution (35-37°C, pH 7.38) that was continuously bubbled with carbogen. The muscle was split at the nerve entry and an innervated strip of muscle tissue was spread out and fixed with small steel needles on a ribbed block of silicon rubber. To prevent nerve stimulation from eliciting muscle fibre action potentials and contractions the tissue was pinched with a pair of small tweezers, beginning at the distal ends of the strip ('cut fibres', cf. Gertler & Robbins, 1978). Intracellular recordings were obtained with glass microelectrodes (4-10 MΩ) filled with 3M KCl. Recordings were rejected if: (i) the initial membrane potential was less negative than -50 mV; (ii) membrane potential decreased by more than 20% from its initial value. All penetrations were from fibre regions with visible miniature end-plate potentials. Full-size EPPs were elicited by electrical stimulation of the nerve (0.1 ms pulses). Recordings from penetrated muscle fibres included: (a) five initial single EPPs (stimulation at 0.5 Hz); (b) EPPs obtained during fatigue-test stimulation of *either* 40-Hz bursts of 0.33 sec repeated once a sec during 2 min *or* 80-Hz continuous stimulation during 30 sec; (c) after 1 min rest: five single EPPs.

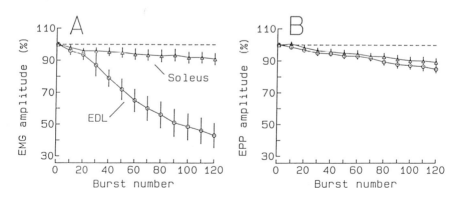

Figure 1. Relative changes (%; means±SE) of EMG and EPP amplitude during 40 Hz fatigue test stimulation (bursts) lasting 2 min. **A** Peak-to-peak sizes of compound action potentials (M waves), as recorded in vivo from 6 Sol and 7 EDL muscles. **B** EPP amplitudes for 12 Sol and 11 EDL muscle fibres, as recorded intracellularly in vitro. Interrupted lines drawn at y = 100%.

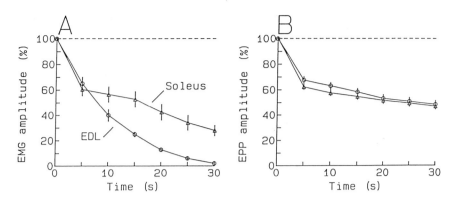

Figure 2. Display as in Fig.1, but for 80-Hz continuous fatigue-test stimulation. **A** From 6 Sol and 6 EDL muscles. **B** From 18 Sol and 13 EDL muscle fibres.

Our results showed that, during either type of fatigue-test stimulation, the mean decline of EPP amplitude was the same for fibres from Sol and EDL (40-Hz test, Fig.1B; 80-Hz test, Fig.2B). Following either test procedure, 1 min rest was sufficient for a full post-stimulation recovery of EPP amplitude.

The mean initial EPP size was significantly greater for Sol (14.6 ± 3.8 (S.D.) mV, n=27) than for EDL (10.1 ± 3.8 mV, n=20; t test, $P<0.001$). With regard to the EPP time course or the resting membrane potential (average -57 mV), no significant differences were found between Sol and EDL.

Our results indicate that the differences in EMG depression between Sol and EDL (Figs.1A, 2A) were not caused by differences in the fatigue-test associated decline of EPP sizes (Figs.1B, 2B). The differences in EMG depression might still have been caused by a greater safety of neuromuscular transmission for Sol than for EDL if the initial amount of excess EPP size, above the threshold for action potential initiation, were normally greater for Sol than for EDL. Alternatively (or additionally), the differences in EMG depression (Figs.1A, 2A) might have been caused by differences in a fatigue-associated decline of the amplitude of sarcolemmal action potentials.

In the intracellular end-plate studies of Gertler & Robbins (1978) and Lev-Tov (1987), certain differences in EPP-behaviour were indeed observed between Sol and EDL. However, the test stimulation procedures of these investigations were different from the present ones. Still, the observations of Gertler and Robbins (1978) on curarized fibres seem consistent with the present findings; in their cases a continuous 40-Hz stimulation (200 pulses) caused a depression of about the same relative magnitude in Sol and EDL (quantum content down to 20.7% of initial value in curarized Sol and to 21.9% in curarized EDL; in 'cut fibres', however, depression was to 42.7% in Sol and to 32.2% in EDL). The study of Lev-Tov (1987) differs fundamentally from the present one by specifically concerning the *potentiating* EPP behaviour that becomes revealed when quantum content is kept low.

References

Enoka RM, Rankin LL, Stuart DG & Volz KA (1989). Fatigability of rat hindlimb muscle: associations between electromyogram and force during a fatigue test. *Journal of Physiology* **408**, 251-270.

Gertler RA & Robbins N (1978). Differences in neuromuscular transmission in red and white muscles. *Brain Research* **142**, 160-164.

Lev-Tov A (1987). Junctional transmission in fast- and slow-twitch mammalian motor units. *Journal of Neurophysiology* **57**, 660-671.

Section III

Long Term Processes: Usage Related Plasticity; Ageing; Damage

Measurement and biochemical correlates of power fatigue resistance in transformed skeletal muscles

S. Salmons, J.C. Jarvis, C.N. Mayne and H. Sutherland

British Heart Foundation Skeletal Muscle Assist Research Group, Department of Human Anatomy and Cell Biology, P.O. Box 147, University of Liverpool, L69 3BX, U.K.

Most people can define fatigue, but what is fatigue resistance? The question needs answering, for clinical as well as scientific reasons. Functional grafts of skeletal muscle are already being used to construct new sphincters and to provide assistance to a failing heart. These new surgical approaches depend on 'conditioning' the skeletal muscle with long-term electrical stimulation so that it does not fatigue when called upon to perform its task continuously. In these circumstances, it is important to define 'fatigue resistance' in relation to the work the muscle is required to sustain.

A muscle will be resistant to fatigue if it can supply, on a continuous basis, sufficient ATP to meet the prevailing energy costs of contraction. These costs derive mainly from the cyclic turnover of chemical bonds between actin and myosin and the transport of calcium between intracellular compartments. During the conditioning process, skeletal muscle is believed to acquire more favourable bioenergetics for sustained contraction as a result of changes both in the isoforms of myosin and in the kinetics of the release and uptake of calcium. At the same time, sustained production of ATP becomes possible through an increase in the capacity of oxidative pathways, particularly those involved in the breakdown of fatty acids. There is an associated increase in blood supply and mitochondrial volume. As a result, ATP production can match even extreme increases in ATP utilization (Clark et al. 1988; Mayne et al. 1991a).

Although the fatigue-resistant nature of conditioned muscle has been known for some years (Salmons & Sréter 1976; Hudlicka et al. 1977), the initial observations were made with fatigue tests based on isometric contractions. More recently, we have used a new ergometer apparatus (Jarvis & Salmons 1990) and a new experimental protocol to investigate the endurance of muscles under conditions in which they perform external work.

Physiological and biochemical measurement of power fatigue

Force-velocity curves were obtained from rabbit tibialis anterior muscles over the full physiological range of shortening velocity by the method of iso-velocity release. Measurements were digitized and processed, and the data plotted as force-velocity and power-velocity curves. For each muscle, single contractions were elicited at the velocity for maximum power (V_{opt}); activation was long enough to produce the full range of movement (19.5 mm). The work done by the muscles was then calculated as the area under the force-time curve (active–passive) multiplied by the velocity.

Since the work performed by the conditioned and control muscles in a single contraction was very different, the fatigue resistance of the two muscles was tested as follows. The muscle masses were estimated from our previous data. Repeated contractions were then set up at a frequency calculated to produce an initial power output, from each muscle, of 10 W/kg wet weight. The power output was monitored over a period of about 4 hours. At the end of the test the muscles were removed, weighed and snap-frozen for subsequent morphometric and biochemical analysis. The actual power output per kg used in the subsequent analyses was calculated using the measured muscle mass, rather than that estimated during the experiment.

After 2 weeks of continuous stimulation at 10 Hz, the conditioned muscle was able to maintain the initial power output over 5 hours, whereas the contralateral control muscle fatigued progressively. After 8 weeks, the instantaneous power output of the stimulated muscle was lower because of reductions in force and contractile speed. The initial working rate of 10 W/kg therefore represented 20% of the maximum instantaneous power output for the stimulated muscle, as against 2.5% for the control muscle. Nevertheless, the stimulated muscle could maintain this level of working better than the control muscle. After 12 weeks, 10 W/kg was close to the maximum for the stimulated muscles: the duty cycle was about 50%, and the muscles were so slow that any further decrease in speed would not have allowed them to relax fully between contractions. These muscles had very high fatigue resistance—probably higher than that of naturally-occurring slow muscle. The homogeneity of muscles stimulated for these long periods is such that the whole-muscle properties probably reflect quite closely those of the constituent fibres.

We reasoned that it should be possible to measure fatigue resistance as the sustained working rate, in W/kg, at which ATP production is just able to keep pace with ATP consumption. To test this, we removed small samples from control muscles during a variety of stimulation régimes and analysed their metabolite composition by HPLC.

During the first 15 min of stimulation we observed the fall in ATP and PCr, and the corresponding rise in creatine and IMP, that are synonymous with fatigue. However, this was followed by spontaneous recovery of these metabolites to control levels, despite a continuing profound force fatigue (Mayne et al. 1991b). This phenomenon, which has been observed by others, may be due to a block in excitation-contraction coupling. Since force fatigue can occur in this way without exhaustion of intracellular ATP, metabolite levels do not provide an unambiguous indicator of fatigue.

Myosin isoforms and fatigue resistance

Recently, we have been comparing the effects of stimulation at 10 Hz and 2.5 Hz. Both the rate and extent of transformation were less when the muscles were stimulated at 2.5 Hz. Mechanical, biochemical and histochemical data were consistent with transformation of the 2B fibre type population of these muscles to the 2A type. Muscles stimulated at 2.5 Hz were significantly faster and more powerful than those stimulated at 10 Hz, yet they proved just as resistant to fatigue when tested under the conditions already described. Since there was no evidence that stimulation at 2.5 Hz for periods up to 12 weeks had induced synthesis of Type 1 myosin isoforms, we conclude that changes in the bioenergetics of contraction associated with myosin transitions are not a major factor in the development of fatigue resistance.

Conclusions

1. Fatigue resistance should be measured in terms of the sustainable rate of performing external work.
2. Fatigue can occur in the presence of normal levels of energy metabolites.
3. Changes in myosin isoforms appear to be much less important in relation to fatigue resistance than changes in blood flow, metabolism and, possibly, the energy costs of calcium transport.

References

Clark BJ III, Acker MA, McCully K, Subramanian HV, Hammond RL, Salmons S, Chance B & Stephenson LW (1988). In vivo ^{31}P-NMR spectroscopy of chronically stimulated canine skeletal muscle. *American Journal of Physiology* **254**, C258-66.

Hudlicka O, Brown M, Cotter M, Smith M & Vrbová G (1977). The effect of long-term stimulation of fast muscles on their blood flow, metabolism and ability to withstand fatigue. *Pflügers Archives* **369**, 141-149.

Jarvis JC & Salmons S (1990). An electrohydraulic apparatus for the measurement of static and dynamic properties of rabbit muscles. *Journal of Applied Physiology* **70**, 938-941.

Mayne CN, Anderson WA, Hammond RL, Eisenberg BR, Stephenson LW & Salmons S (1991a). Correlates of fatigue resistance in canine skeletal muscle stimulated electrically for up to one year. *American Journal of Physiology* **261**, C259-70.

Mayne CN, Jarvis JC & Salmons S (1991b) Dissociation between metabolite levels and force fatigue in the early stages of stimulation-induced transformation of mammalian skeletal muscle. *Basic & Applied Myology* **1**, 63-70.

Salmons S & Sréter FA (1976). Significance of impulse activity in the transformation of skeletal muscle type. *Nature* **263**, 30-34.

Motor unit heterogeneity with respect to speed and fatiguability in cat muscles after chronic stimulation or paralysis

T. Gordon, M.C. Pattullo, V.F. Rafuse

Department of Pharmacology and Division of Neuroscience, 525 Heritage Medical Research Center, Faculty of Medicine, Edmonton, Alberta, T6G 2S2.

Chronic stimulation of fast-twitch muscles in rabbit (Salmons & Vrbova, l969; reviewed by Pette & Vrbova, 1985) and cat (Eerbeek et al., 1984; reviewed by Kernell & Eerbeek,1989) has been shown to change contractile properties toward those of slow muscles. Activation with total daily amounts of activity of > 30%, 5% and <0.5% of the day, corresponding roughly with the activity of slow (S), fast-fatigue resistant (FR) and fast fatiguable (FF) units, appeared to convert the muscle contraction characteristics toward those of the predicted motor unit (MU) type (Eerbeek et al., 1984; Kernell et al., 1987a,b; Westgaard & Lomo, 1988). If activity causes complete conversion, the prediction would be that all MUs in the stimulated muscles would become homogeneous in their properties. We therefore asked 2 questions: 1) what are the effects and the time course of increasing or decreasing activity on muscle speed and endurance? and 2) do MUs become homogeneous with respect to force, speed and endurance as predicted if activity converts muscles rather than modulates their properties within an adaptive range (Ausoni et al., 1990; Westgaard & Lomo, 1988).

Experimental methods

Silastic cuffs containing 3 stainless steel electrodes were aseptically implanted unilaterally around the nerve to medial gastrocnemius (MG) muscle in 13 adult cats (3-4 Kg), under pentobarbitone (60mg/Kg; i.p.) anaesthetic. A bipolar pad electrode was sutured to the fascia of MG muscle and the wires of all electrodes led out through the skin for 1) connection to a portable stimulator mounted on a basket carried on the cat's back for chronic stimulation and 2) for connection to external stimulators and amplifiers for regular recording of evoked EMG and isometric force.

The cats were divided into 2 groups. In group A (n=7), MG muscle was stimulated supramaximally at 20Hz with a 50% duty cycle (2.5 sec on, 2.5 sec off) for 6 to 34 weeks. In group B (n=6), the spinal cord was hemisected at L1 and the right hindlimb deafferented extradurally (L1-S2). Evoked EMG and isometric muscle force were measured at weekly intervals in both groups under halothane anaesthesia (for details see Gordon & Stein, 1982a) to monitor changes in force, contractile speed and fatiguability. The fatigue index (FI) for the muscle was calculated as the ratio of force generated at the end and beginning of a 2 minute period of tetanic trains of 13 pulses at 40Hz/1 sec. In a final acute experiment, 6-34 weeks later, all hindlimb muscles other than the MG were denervated and a laminectomy performed under pentobarbitone anesthesia, for isolation and characterization of muscle and single motor unit properties, using criteria described in detail by Gordon & Stein (1982b). Muscles were frozen and 10μm cross-sections were later cut for histochemical classification of muscle fibres (see Gordon et al., 1988). Muscle and motor unit properties were also studied in a third group C (n=6) which did not undergo surgery and provided the control data for comparison.

Results

There was little change in either contractile force or speed in MG paralysed by hemisection and deafferentation but muscle endurance decreased significantly. The mean (± S.E) tetanic force of

6 muscles which were paralysed for an average of 236 ± 45 days was 62 ± 5 N, as compared to 69 ± 6 N in contralateral control muscles. The twitch contraction time (CT) of 46 ± 2 ms was similar to that of the normal muscles, 50 ± 1.7 ms. FI was significantly less in paralysed muscles (cf. 0.25 ± 0.07 and 0.02 ± 0.01). There was a corresponding increase in the proportion of FF units (51% as compared with 31%) and fast glycolytic (FG) muscle fibres (58% as compared with 45%) which accounted for the decline in FI of the whole muscle. The relative number of S units and slow oxidative fibres (S0) of 28% did not change. Examination of a large population of MUs (n=180) showed that paralysed muscles contain the normal heterogeneous population with a wide range of unit CT and FI (Fig. 1).

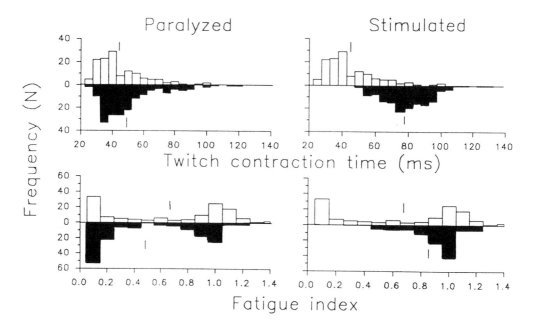

Figure 1. Comparisons of frequency distributions of twitch contraction times and fatigue indices of motor units sampled from paralysed (Group A) and chronically stimulated (Group B) cat MG muscles (solid histograms) with normal (Group C) muscles (open histograms). Mean values are shown as vertical bars. Further details are provided in the text.

In contrast, the contractile force and speed declined in the stimulated muscles and the endurance increased, as previously shown (Eerbeek et al., 1984; Kernell et al., 1987a,b). At six weeks, muscle force decreased (47 ± 5 N as compared to 63 ± 8 N in 3 cats) with relatively little change in CT or FI (cf 48 ± 2 ms and 51 ± 3 ms, CT; 0.32 ± 0.01 and 0.25 ± 0.05, FI). Over longer periods (158 ± 30 days, n=4), muscle twitch CT and FI increased significantly from 46 ± 2 ms to 96 ± 4 and 0.25 ± 0.07 to 0.7 ± 0.16, respectively.
There was a corresponding increase in mean CT and FI in isolated MUs: 78 ± 1 and 0.85 ± 0.02 in 168 MUs in 4 stimulated muscles, as compared with 43 ± 1 and 0.64 ± 0.04 in 134 units in 6 normal muscles (vertical bars in Fig. 1). However, the range of CT and FI was NOT reduced to the range of normal S units, as predicted for complete transformation of the MG from fast-twitch to slow-twitch. Comparison of the frequency histograms for MUs in normal and stimulated muscles shows that twitch CT is increased after stimulation but covers as large a range as normal. The normal bimodal distribution of FI becomes unimodal but the range is not confined to values above 0.75 as expected for complete conversion of MUs to non-fatiguable S MUs (see Kernell & Eerbeek, 1989).

Discussion

Although it has generally been accepted since the classical work of Sarah Tower (1937) that paralysed muscles undergo atrophic changes, we find surprisingly little change in properties of the paralysed cat MG muscle, other than a significant decrease in muscle endurance (see also Mayer et al., 1984; Pierotti et al., 1992, Munson et al., 1986). Similar findings have been observed in ankle flexor muscles (Kernell et al., 1987a,b). For the many different models of disuse which have been studied, effects of reduced muscle activity vary widely but there is general agreement that disused muscles become more fatiguable (Roy et al., 1991).

Results of slowing of fast-twitch muscles, increase in contractile speed of slow- twitch muscles, and conversion of muscle fibre types after cross-reinnervation or chronic stimulation have been interpreted as a "switch" from one phenotype to another, consistent with the appropriate expression of slow or fast isoforms of regulatory and contractile proteins and metabolic enzymes in the converted muscles (Vrbova et al., 1978; Pette & Vrbova, 1985). However, recent findings which show a significant increase in the number of muscle fibres expressing more than one isoform of these proteins, despite a change in muscle properties and muscle fibre types, suggest that muscle properties may be adapted rather than converted (reviewed by Pette & Staron, 1990). From studies that recognise differences in myotube phenotype prior to innervation, which are subsequently modulated by innervation during development (Miller & Stockdale, 1987), the possibility arises that intrinsic properties of muscle fibres are modulated by neural activity rather than converted: a plasticity which is limited within an adaptive range preset by intrinsic properties (see Ausoni et al., 1990). Analysis of motor unit properties after synchronous activation of all MUs in chronically stimulated muscles shows that the MU population is NOT homogeneous with respect to force, contractile speed and fatiguability which is the result predicted if activity CONVERTED muscle properties to that of slow MUs. Rather stimulation led to slowing of ALL MUs and increased their endurance, consistent with a modulation of properties. Thus, apparent conversion of fast-twitch to slow-twitch muscles by chronic stimulation is not simply a "switch" from a fast-phenotype to slow but rather a modulation of the MU population within an adaptive range, possibly preset by intrinsic mechanisms which are independent of activity.

Acknowledgements

This work was supported by the Medical Research Council and Network of Centres of Excellence, Canada.

References

Ausoni S, Gorza L, Schiaffino S, Gundersen K & Lomo T (1990). Expression of myosin heavy chain isoforms in stimulated fast and slow rat muscles. *J. Neurosci.* **10**, 153- 160.

Eerbeek O, Kernell D & Verhey BA (1984). Effects of fast and slow patterns of tonic stimulation on contractile properties of fast muscles in the cat. *J. Physiol.* **352,** 773- 790.

Gordon T & Stein RB (1982a). Reorganization of motor-unit properties in reinnervated muscles of the cat. *J. Neurophysiol.* **48**, 1175-1190.

Gordon T & Stein RB (1982b). Time course and extent of recovery in reinnervated motor units of cat triceps surae muscles. *J. Physiol.* **323,** 307-323.

Gordon T, Thomas CK, Stein RB & Erdebil S (1988). Comparison of physiological and histochemical properties of motor units following cross-reinnervation of antagonistic muscles in the cat hindlimb. *J. Neurophysiol.* **60**, 365-378.

Kernell D & Eerbeek O (1989). Physiological effects of different patterns of chronic stimulation on muscle properties. In *Neuromuscular Stimulation.* Eds, Rose FC & Jones R . Demos Publications, New York, USA.

Kernell D , Eerbeek O, Verhey BA & Donselaar Y (1987a). Effects of physiological amounts of high-and low-rate chronic stimulation of fast-twitch muscle of the cat hindlimb. I. Speed- and force-related properties. *J. Neurophysiol.* **58**, 598-613.

Kernell D, Donselaar Y & Eerbeek O (1987b). Effects of physiological amounts of high- and low-rate chronic stimulation of fast-twitch muscle of the cat hindlimb. II. Endurance-related properties. *J. Neurophysiol.* **58**, 614-627.

Mayer RF, Burke RE, Toop J, Walmsley B & Hodgson JA (1984). The effect of spinal cord transection on motor units in cat medial gastrocnemius muscles. *Muscle & Nerve* **7**, 23-31.

Miller JB & Stockdale FE (1987). What muscle cells know that nerves don't tell them. *TINS* **10**, 325-329.

Munson JB, Foehring RC, Lofton SA, Zengel JE & Sypert GW (1986). Plasticity of medial gastrocnemius motor units following cordotomy in the cat. *J. Neurophysiol.* **55**, 619-634.

Pette P & Staron RS (1990). Cellular and molecular diversities of mammalian skeletal muscle fibres. *Rev. Physiol. Biochem. Pharmacol.* **116**, 1-16.

Pette D & Vrbova G (1985). Invited review: neural control of phenotypic expression in mammalian muscle fibres. *Muscle & Nerve* **8**, 676-689.

Pierotti DJ, Roy RR, Bodine-Fowler SC, Hodgson JA & Edgerton VR (1992). Mechanical and morphologic properties of chronically inactive cat tibialis anterior motor units. *J. Physiol.* (in press).

Roy RR, Baldwin FM & Edgerton VR (1991). The plasticity of skeletal muscle: effects of neuromuscular activity. *Exercise & Sports Sc. Rev.* **19**, 269-312.

Salmons S & Vrbova G (1969). The influence of activity on some activity on some contractile characteristics of mammalian fast and slow muscles. *J. Physiol.* **201**, 535-549.

Tower SS (1937). Function and structure in the chronically isolated lumbo-sacral spinal cord of the dog. *J. Comp. Neurol.* **67**, 109-131.

Vrbova G, Gordon T & Jones R (1978). *Nerve-Muscle Interaction.* Chapman & Hall, London.

Westgaard RH & Lomo T (1988). Control of contractile properties within adaptive ranges of impulse activity in the rat. *J. Neurosci.* **8**, 4415-4426.

Muscle disuse enhances performance of rat medial gastrocnemius on a standard fatigue test in situ

P. Gardiner, M. Favron, and P. Corriveau

Département d'éducation physique, Université de Montréal, C.P. 6128, Succ. A, Montréal, Québec, Canada H3C 3J7

The effects of decreased neuromuscular usage on the fatigability of the affected muscles remains controversial. The model of disuse induced by blockage of motor nerve impulses by chronic nerve superfusion with the sodium channel blocker tedrodotoxin (TTX) provides an unequivocal means of addressing this issue, since it evokes complete motoneurone silence which is quickly reversed when TTX is removed. In the present study, we examined fatigue resistance of a rat ankle extensor subjected to 2 weeks of complete disuse, using an in situ fatigue regimen which is frequently used to distinguish motor unit types in cat and rat muscles. We have found that previously disused muscles are more fatigue resistant, and perform more contractile work, in spite of severe fiber atrophy and a decreased activity of the mitochondrial marker enzyme succinate dehydrogenase (SDH) in muscle fibers.

Female Sprague-Dawley rats (225 g) had one hindlimb paralyzed for 2 weeks by blocking sciatic nerve impulses chronically with TTX, using a surgically-implanted constant-delivery system described previously (St-Pierre et al.1988). After 14 days of paralysis, isometric in situ contractile properties of the left medial gastrocnemius in response to sciatic nerve stimulation were recorded from anesthetized animals. After recording twitch and tetanic (200 Hz) responses, fatigue resistance was monitored for 5 minutes, using the stimulation protocol described by Burke et al. (1973). Muscles were subsequently frozen at rest length in melting isopentane, sections were cut at -20°C, and treated for the quantitative measurement of SDH activity (Martin et al.1985).

As in previous experiments (St-Pierre et al.1988), the main effect of TTX-induced disuse included decreased maximum tetanic force (by 70%) which was attributable to fiber atrophy (65%). In addition, twitch/tetanic ratios were significantly elevated after disuse (from .18±.01 to .50±.02). In response to the Burke fatigue protocol (Fig. 1A), previously disused muscles began contractions at a higher percentage of maximum tetanic force (68%) than control muscles, and showed less potentiation of forces during the first 15 seconds. At all time intervals up to 5 minutes, disused muscles generated significantly ($p<.01$) higher relative forces than controls. Fatigue index (measured as the force drop relative to peak response) was significantly higher after 2 and 4 minutes for disused muscles, indicating increased fatigue resistance in spite of generating higher forces relative to maximum tetanic force, compared to controls (Fig. 1B). As a post hoc consideration, we added a control group in which fatigue resistance was measured in response to stimulation at a frequency which would result in initial high relative forces similar to those seen for the disused muscles (75 Hz, 100 ms, once per s). In the latter, fatigue resistance was similar to that seen in the control muscles subjected to the Burke procedure. In contrast to the greater performance of the disused muscles during the fatigue protocol, the activity of the mitochondrial enzyme SDH was significantly reduced (by 26%) in individual muscle fibers (Fig. 1C).

The results support previous demonstrations with the models of suspension hypokinesia (Fell et al.1985) and immobilization (Robinson et al.1991) that muscle disuse enhances fatigue resistance. The latter occurred in spite of reduced activity of a mitochondrial marker enzyme, thus substantiating the hypothesis (Hamm et al.1988) that fatigue resistance and muscle oxidative potential may be coincidentally related among the various motor unit types. The altered frequency-tension relationship and the lack of potentiation in disused muscles suggests that calcium mobilization mechanisms are involved. Lower mitochondrial content may reduce calcium uptake by these organelles during fatigue, maintaining calcium availability for continued uptake and release (Tate et al.1978). This model is currently being studied to determine the factors limiting contractile performance in this altered muscular state.

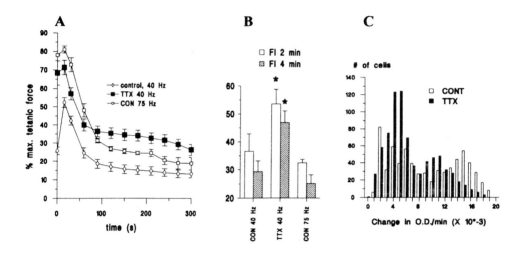

Figure 1.(A) Force decrements of the three groups during the fatigue protocol. (B) Fatigue index. (C) Histogram of fiber SDH activities for control and TTX muscles.

Burke R, Levine D, Tsairis p & Zajac F (1973). Physiological types and histochemical profiles in motor units of the cat gastrocnemius. *Journal of Physiology* **234**, 723-748.

Fell R, Gladden B, Steffen J & Musacchia X (1985). Fatigue and contraction of slow and fast muscles in hypokinetic/hypodynamic rats. *Journal of Applied Physiology* **58**, 65-69.

Hamm T, Nemeth P, Solanki L, Gordon D, Reinking R & Stuart D (1988). Association between biochemical and physiological properties in single motor units. *Muscle & Nerve* **11**,245-254.

Martin T, Vailas A, Durivage J, Edgerton V & Castleman K (1985). Quantitative histochemical determination of muscle enzymes : biochemical verification. *Journal of Histochemistry and Cytochemistry* **33**, 1053-1059.

Robinson G, Enoka R & Stuart D (1991). Immobilization-induced changes in motor unit force and fatigability in the cat. *Muscle & Nerve* **14**, 563-573.

St-Pierre D, Leonard D, Houle R & Gardiner P (1988). Recovery from tetrodotoxin -induced disuse and the influence of daily exercise. *Experimental Neurology* **101**, 327-346.

Tate C, Bonner H & Leslie S (1978). Calcium uptake in skeletal muscle mitochondria.*European Journal of Applied Physiology* **39**, 111-122.

Fatigue in hypertrophied rat m.plantaris: age, capillarization and fibre type effects

H. Degens, Z. Turek and R.A. Binkhorst

Dept. of Physiology, University of Nijmegen, P.O. Box 9101, 6500 HB Nijmegen, The Netherlands.

This presentation is part of a study concerning age and hypertrophy effects on capillarization, fibre type composition and functioning of rat m. plantaris, in which also fatigue was studied. Fatigue is defined as a decline of force during repeated isometric contractions at a constant stimulation pattern. We investigated if relations between fibre type composition and capillarization at one side and fatigue on the other side could be found in our material and if these relations were modulated by ageing and compensatory hypertrophy.

Materials and Methods

Used were female Wistar rats of 5, 13 and 25 months of age at the time of the experiments. Hypertrophy was obtained by denervation of synergists (Binkhorst, 1969). Six weeks later isometric contraction measurements were done and fatigue resistance tested by the protocol described by Burke et al (1973). A Fatigue Index (FAT) was defined as Peak force of a tetanic contraction 2 min after strongest contraction divided by peak force in strongest contraction (Fatigue-Index A, Kernell et al.1987). Thereafter transverse sections of the muscle were cut on a cryostat. Fibres were classified as type I or II based on their ATP-ase staining and subclassified into oxidative (IIa) and Glycolytic (IIb) from SDH staining. Capillaries were depicted by combined staining for Alkaline Phosphatase and Dipeptidyl Peptidase IV (Degens et al.1992). Determined was the CD (Capillary Density) as number of capillaries per mm^2 tissue and the % area occupied by a fibre type of the total cross-sectional muscle area occupied by fibres. Age and hypertrophy effects were tested by applying an ANOVA. Pearson Correlations coefficients were calculated between CD and % area of fibre types as independent variables and the FAT as dependent variable for each age group for both hypertrophied and control muscles. Values are mean ± SEM. Tested was at a significance level of $P < 0.05$.

Results

The FAT was significantly higher in 13 months (0.45 ± 0.02; n=33) than 5 months old muscles (0.36 ± 0.02; n=32) but did not differ significantly from that of 25 months old muscles (0.37 ± 0.04; n=28). Compensatorily hypertrophied muscles showed a significantly higher FAT than controls at all ages. They also showed a decreased % area IIb. In figure 1 the FAT is plotted against the % area of type IIb fibres (Fig.1A) and the CD (Fig.1B) respectively. No significant correlations between the FAT and % area I, % area IIb and/or CD were found in neither group, although the FAT tended to be negatively related to the % area IIb (Fig.1A). Even when all data were pooled and in addition ultiple correlations were calculated no significant relations appeared between the FAT as dependent variable and % area I, % area IIb and CD as independent variables.

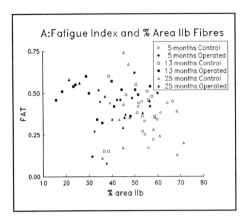 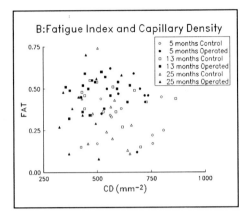

Figure 1. A.Fatigue index (FAT) and % area IIb fibres (%IIb): r=-0.20; P=0.08; n=72. B.FAT and Capillary Density: r=-0.12; P=0.27; n=79.

Discussion

The results of the present study indicate that there is no significant relation between the areal fraction of glycolytic fibres and Capillary density on one side and Fatigue resistance as assessed by applying the "Burke Test" on the other side in whole muscle. In addition other studies showed that changes in SDH activity were not tightly coupled to changes in FAT (Kernell et al.1987). This suggests that the occurrence of fatigue is probably not tightly related to the oxidative capacity and oxygen supply, but probably more to e.g. an impaired excitation contraction coupling.

References

Binkhorst RA (1969) The effect of training on some isometric contraction characteristics of a fast muscle. *Pflügers Archiv* **309**, 193-202.

Burke RE, Levine DN, Tsairis P & Zajac FE (1973) Physiological types and histochemical profiles in motor units of the cat gastrocnemius. *Journal of Physiology (London)* **234**, 723-748.

Degens H, Turek Z, Hoofd LJC, van 't Hof MA & Binkhorst RA (1992) The relationship between capillarization and fibre types in the compensatorily hypertrophied m. plantaris of the rat. *Journal of Anatomy* (Accepted).

Kernell D, Donselaar Y & Eerbeek O (1987) Effects of physiological amounts of high- and low-rate chronic stimulation on fast-twitch muscle of the cat hindlimb. Endurance related properties. *Journal of Neurophysiology* **58**, 614-627.

Fatigue paradox in the elderly

M.V. Narici, M. Bordini and P. Cerretelli

Reparto di Fisiologia del Lavoro Muscolare, Istituto di Tecnologie Biomediche Avanzate, Consiglio Nazionale delle Ricerche, via Ampère 56, 20131, Milan, Italy

Ageing is characterized by a sequence of events leading to a functional reduction of a chain of systems. Among the various tissues and organs affected by this process skeletal muscle undergoes functional and structural changes (Larsson 1978) that are likely to influence the quality of life of the individual. This study was therefore conducted with the aim of investigating the extent and onset of the changes of human skeletal muscle function induced by the process of ageing.

Experimental methods

Both voluntary and electrically evoked isometric contractions of the adductor pollicis muscle (AP) were studied in seventy healthy male subjects aged 20-91yr, 10 for each decade. After warming of the hand and forearm in hot water ($\geq 40°C$) for 5 min, maximum isometric voluntary contraction (MVC) of the AP was measured and the highest value out of three trials was chosen. Electrical stimulation of the AP was carried out at the wrist with supramaximal 50 μs square-wave impulses as described by Edwards et al. (1977). The frequency-force relationship was determined by a train of impulses at 1, 10, 20, 30 and 50 Hz for 2 s each and expressing force values as the percentage of the force at 50 Hz. Maximum relaxation rate (MRR) was measured from the differential of the force signal after stimulation of the muscle for 1 s at 30 Hz and was expressed as the percent decrease in force over 10 ms. Isometric endurance was assessed during a 30-s stimulation at 30 Hz and was defined as the percentage of the final force over the initial force.

Statistics.
ANOVA was used to determine wether the age factor had any significant effect on MVC, frequency-force relationship, MRR and endurance. To locate differences between means the Tukey test of critical differences was applied, significance was set at the 5% level. All data are reported as means±SE.

Results

Isometric MVC was quite well mantained up the age of 59 yr but thereafter showed a significant decline ($p < 0.001 - 0.05$, Tukey test) and by the eight decade had dropped to 42.4% of its original (2nd decade) value (Fig 1). The 10/50, 20/50 and 30/50 Hz force ratios of the age group > 80 yr were significantly higher than those of the 20-29 and 30-39 yr groups ($p < 0.05 - 0.001$). A shift to the left of the frequency/force relationship was observed in the oldest age group (Fig 2) and fusion was virtually complete at 30 Hz as compared to 50 Hz in the two youngest groups (20-29 and 30-39 yr). MRR similarly to MVC, did not show any significant deterioration prior to the age of 59 yr after which the rate of decline became significantly faster ($p < 0.05 - 0.001$). From the second to the eight decade it decreased by of 48.7% (Fig 3). Isometric endurance showed a paradoxical, linear increase with age ($p < 0.001$, Fig 4) and from the second to the eigth decade the increase was of 25.5%.

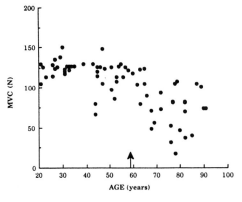

Figure 1. Individual values of maximum voluntary contraction (MVC) force from 20 to 91 yr. Arrow , age after which changes in MVC become significant (Tukey test).

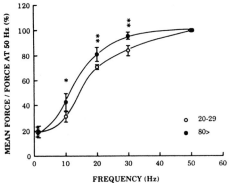

Figure 2. Frequency-force curves for youngest (20-29 yr) and eldest (>80 yr) groups (means ±SE). Group from 30 to 39 yr not shown, because it was not statistically different from 20- to 29-yr group. Significance of Tukey test : * P < 0.05 ; **P < 0.001

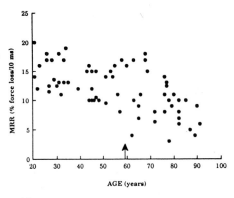

Figure 3. Individual values of maximum relaxation rate (MRR) from 20 to 91 yr. Arrow, age after which changes in MRR become significant (Tukey test).

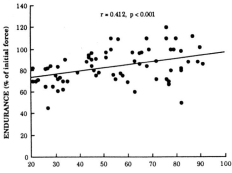

Figure 4. Individual values of isometric endurance from 20 to 91 yr. Correletion coefficient (r) and probability (P) refer to fit of data points in linear regression equation.

(reprinted with permission from
    Narici et al, 1991)

Fatigue paradox in the elderly

Discussion

These findings show that with ageing skeletal muscle becomes weaker, slower, is tetanized at lower fusion frequencies but appears paradoxically more resistant to static fatigue. These changes are probably related to structural alterations of the neuro-muscular system. Muscle atrophy for instance, which may originate from progressive disuse and from the denervation of motor units following axonal degeneration, is probably one of the main causes for the decrease in MVC. This process however, seems to affect type II fibres to a greater extent and leads to a proportionate increase in the relative composition of type I fibres. As these fibres have lower fusion frequencies than type II fibres, an increase in their proportion may concur to the left shift of the force/frequency curve. This effect may also be related to the longer relaxation times of type I fibres than those of type II. An increase in relaxation time would lead not only to a decrease in MRR but also to tetanization at lower frequencies. The reinnervation process of denervated type II fibres by sprouting axons of motor neurons of slow-twitch motor units (Gardiner et al. 1987) and damage to the sarcoplasmic reticulum may also account for the slowing down of muscle (Klitgaard et al. 1989). The paradoxical increase in isometric endurance may be consequential to the relative increase in the proportion of the more fatigue-resistant type I fibres but may also be related to the force potentiation resulting from the slower relaxation. It may be thus concluded that with ageing, despite the decrease in force, the slowing down of muscle and loss of anaerobic muscle fibres may act as "preservation mechanisms" for the maintenance of force during prolongued, static contractions.

References

Edwards RHT, Young A, Hosking GP & Jones DA (1977). Human skeletal muscle function: description of tests and normal values. *Clinical Science and Molecular Medicine* **52**, 283-290.

Gardiner P, Michel R, Olha A & Pettigrew F (1987). Force and fatiguability of sprouting motor units in partially denervated rat plantaris. *Experimental Brain Research* **66**, 597-606.

Klitgaard H, Ausoni S & Damiani E (1989). Sarcoplasmic reticulum of human skeletal muscle: age-related changes and effect of training. *Acta Physiologica Scandinavica* **137**, 23-31.

Larsson L (1978). Morphological and functional characteristics of the ageing skeletal muscle in man. A cross-sectional study. *Acta Physiologica Scandinavica Supplement* **457**, 1-36.

Narici MV, Borelini M & P. Cerretelli (1991). Effect of ageing on human adductor pollicis muscle function. *Journal of Applied Physiology* **71** : 1277-1281.

A single training session affects exercise-induced muscle damage in the rat

P.J. Bosman, W.A.F. Balemans, G.J. Amelink and P.R. Bär

Research Laboratory Neurology, University Hospital Utrecht, Heidelberglaan 100
3584 CX Utrecht, The Netherlands

Exercise can cause transient damage to skeletal muscle, as has been demonstrated by numerous studies in humans (Ebbeling and Clarkson 1989) and in animals (after eccentric exercise: Armstrong et al. 1983, after concentric exercise: Amelink and Bär 1986). Damage is evidenced by elevations of serum enzymes such as CK as well as by histological signs of muscle damage. In humans this is often accompanied by muscle soreness and impaired muscle function (Bär et al. 1990).

A single bout of exercise can protect the muscle against damage caused by a subsequent work. This rapid adaptation is especially notable in humans after eccentric exercise (Ebbeling and Clarkson 1989). We describe the effect of one bout of exercise studied in a level (concentric) running rat model, on damage caused by a second, identical exercise session. Plasma CK activity was used as a marker for muscle damage. As we have shown before, most of the rise of the CK activity after exercise in this model is indeed derived from muscle (Amelink et al. 1988).

Experimental Methods

In the experiment 13 male Wistar rats (215 g ± 9) were used. A jugular vein cannula, reaching into the hart, was implanted one week before exercise. The rats were subjected to a 2 h level treadmill run at 19 m/min. After the first run the rats were randomly divided into group A (7 rats) and group B (6 rats). Both group A and group B rats were subjected to a second, identical, bout of exercise: group A after 1 day and group B after 6 days. The CK activity in serum was measured before and immediately after exercise.

Statistics

Because of the cannulation repeated blood sampling is possible, so that animals serve as their own controls. For statistical analysis of the data within one session the paired version of the Student's t-test was used, for comparison of data between sessions the unpaired t-test was used.

Results

Figure 1 shows the effect of one bout of exercise on muscle damage caused during a second exercise session 1 day or 6 days later. After the first bout the serum CK activity had increased significantly from 57 ± 13 to 123 ± 27 U/l (mean ± standard deviation, $p < 0.01$).

After 24 h, the resting CK activity (group A) was significantly lower (38 ± 5 vs 57 ± 13, $p < 0.01$). The increase in CK activity during the second exercise, however, was significantly higher than after the first bout (156 ± 40 and 123 ± 27 U/l resp, $p < 0.05$).

When the second exercise was performed 6 days after the first run (group B), the picture was completely different. Firstly, the CK resting values were not significantly different (54 ± 11 vs 57 ± 13 U/l). Secondly, the increase in CK activity after the second bout is much lower than the increase after the first run (76 ± 30 and 123 ± 27 U/l resp, $p < 0.01$).

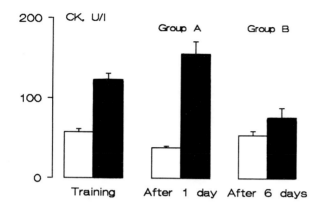

Figure 1. Plasma CK activity before (open bars) and immediately after (closed bars) a 2 h training run in 13 male rats. In 7 rats the exercise was repeated after 1 day (group A), in the remaining 6 rats the exercise was repeated after 6 days (group B).

Discussion

Based on the observation of a lower CK response after exercise in Group B there seems to be a protective effect of a single bout of exercise in rats that run for 2 h on a treadmill. This protection becomes apparent 6 days later. This is in keeping with Armstrong et al. (1983) who found a protective effect of a single bout of exercise when the exercise was repeated 3 days later and CK was measured 48 h after the second exercise. Thus, there is evidence for a rapid adaptation to exercise-induced muscle damage in rats after a single bout of exercise.

However, the fact that repeating the exercise regimen 24 h later resulted in an increased CK response points to an increased susceptibility to exercise-induced muscle damage within the first 24 h after exercise, before a protective effect of the first bout is established. Apparently it takes at least 24 h for the rat muscles to adapt. It is not known what entails the rapid adaptation to exercise-induced muscle damage. Rapid changes in passive resistance to stretch of the muscle (membrane) by reinforcement of the cytoskeleton, which is important in exercise-induced muscle damage (Waterman-Storer 1991) or the extracellular matrix (Stauber et al. 1990) could be responsible, as well as other e.g. metabolic factors.

References

Amelink GJ, Bär PR (1986) Exercise-induced muscle protein leakage in the rat: Effects of hormonal manipulation. *Journal of the Neurological Sciences* **76**, 61-68

Amelink GJ, Kamp HH, Bär PR (1988) Creatine Kinase isoenzyme profiles after exercise in the rat: Sex-linked differences in leakage of CK-MM. *Pflugers Archive European Journal of Physiology* **412**, 417-421

Armstrong RB, Ogilvie RW, Schwane JA (1983) Eccentric exercise-induced injury to rat skeletal muscle. *Journal of Applied Physiology* **54**, 80-93

Bär PR, Amelink GJ, Jackson MJ, Jones DA, Bast A (1990) Aspects of exercise-induced muscle-damage. In: *Sports, Medicine and Health* (Hermans GPH, ed.) Elsevier Science Publishers, Amsterdam pp 1143-1148

Ebbeling CB, Clarkson PM (1989) Exercise-induced muscle damage and adaptation. *Sports Medicine* **7**, 207-234

Stauber WT, Fritz VK, Dahlmann B (1990) Extracellular matrix changes following blunt trauma to rat skeletal muscles. *Experimental and Molecular Pathology* **52**, 69-86

Waterman-Storer CM (1991) The cytoskeleton of skeletal muscle: is it affected by exercise? A brief review. *Medicine and Science in Sports and Exercise* **23**, 1240-1249

Is serum CK related to muscular fatigue in long-distance running?

J. M. C. Soares*, J. A. R. Duarte*, H.-J. Appell[§]

* Department of Sport Biology, Faculty of Sport Sciences, University of Porto, Praça Pedro Nunes, 4000 Porto, Portugal.
§ Institute for Experimental Morphology, German Sports University, Cologne.

Elevation in serum levels of creatine-kinase (CK) activity following various forms of exercise are well documented (Hortobágyi & Denaham 1989). Plasma CK activity has been used as an indicator of muscle damage, especially after eccentric exercise (Schwane et al. 1983). Exercise-induced damage has been assessed using changes in motor performance, i.e. muscular fatigue (Clarkson e Tremblay 1988). The mechanisms by which exercise results in loss of functional capacity has not been clearly identified (Appell et al. 1991; Soares et al. 1992). The purpose of the present study was to examine the serum CK in response to 2 long-distance runs during 2 consecutive days.

Material and methods

Nine fully informed, consenting and healthy male long-distance runners (mean age 31.1 yrs) participated in this study. All subjects performed 2 runs of 12 km each at their personal competition intensity during 2 consecutive days. Blood samples were obtained before the first run (B1R), 60 min after the first run (A1R), before the second run (B2R), i.e., 24h after the 1R, 60 min (A2R) and 24h after the 2R (24hA2R). Standard venipuncture techniques were used to obtain samples from the antecubital vein. CK activity was measured enzymatically using a commercial kit (CK NAC Activated, Boehringer).

Statistics.
Differences in CK activity among the different moments of evaluation were tested with ANOVA repeated measures. Post hoc comparison was done with the Scheffe F-Test at an alfa of 5%.

Results

The mean ± SD of the CK activity are shown in Table 1. The results evidenced significant intraindividual differences ($p < 0.001$). The CK activity before the 1R was slightly higher than the normal clinical values and increased significantly 60 min after the 1R. The augmentation after the 1R was more pronounced than the increase observed after the 2R (186.8 vs 110%, respectively).
Among the subjects, two different response patterns were observed, one group showed a low CK response, another showed a high CK response (Figure 1).

Table 1. Creatine-kinase activity (U/l), before and after the two consecutive runs.

	B1R	A1R	B2R	A2R	24h2R
Mean	110.2	205.9*	254.2*	282.3*#	165.2
SD	25.4	58.7	71.4	80.9	39.1

* Significant increase compared to the values B1R. # Significant increase compared to the values A1R.

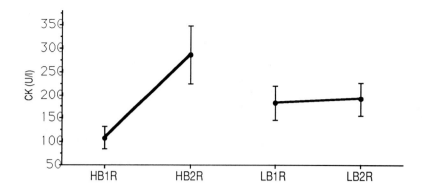

Figure 1. CK activities for the high CK responders before the 1R (HB1R) and for the low CK responders before the 2R (LB2R). Values are means ±SD. All differences are statistically significants, except LB1R to LB2R.

Discussion

Several studies have shown that serum or plasma CK activity increases dramatically after strenous or novel physical exercise (for ref. see Ebbeling & Clarkson 1989) and this increase has provided evidence of exercise-induced muscle damage. A problem with the use of CK in the blood is that CK demonstrates a large intersubject variabilities, particularly for the evaluation of muscle injury (Clarkson et al. 1986). The evaluation of serum CK as a measure for muscle damage shows large intraindividual variabiliy, and three classes of subjects have been described concerning the CK responses to exercise (Clarkson & Ebbeling 1988). The subjects of the present study were attributed to low and high responders, based on expert criteria concerning a cut-off line.

In spite of the large increase in serum CK observed after the 1R, the athletes were able to perform the 2R with high intensity and good performance, suggesting that: (i) either the CK it is not a fiable indicator of muscle damage, (ii) or the muscle damage induced by the 1R (as demonstrated by CK) was not severe enough to impair performance substancially. Recently, however, the prophylatic effect of a single initial exercise bout has been described (Newham et al. 1987). We also assume that the 1R gave some protections to the 2R because the increase observed after the 2R was less pronounced than that registered after the 1R, suggesting a rapid training effect.

The results suggest, that in spite of high serum CK activities, athletes can perform long-distance runs with high intensity. Moreover, a preparative run on a similar track may give certain protection to skeletal muscle.

References

Clarkson PM, Byrnes WC, Gillisson E & Harper E (1986). Adaptation to exercise-induced muscle damage. *Clinical Science* **73**, 383-386

Clarkson PM & Ebbeling C (1988). Investigation of serum creatine kinase variability after muscle-damaging exercise. *Clinical Science* **75**: 257-261

Clarksson PM & Tremblay I (1988). Rapid adaptation to exercise induced muscle damage. *Journal of Applied Physiology* **65**, 1-6

Ebbeling CB & Clarkson PM(1989). Exercise-induced muscle damage and adaptation. *Sports Medicine* **7**: 207-234

Hortobágyi T & Denahan T(1989). Variability in creatine kinase: methodological, exercise, and clinicallyrelated factors. *International Journal of Sports Medicine* **10**, 69-80.

Newham DJ, Jones DA & Clarkson PM (1987). Repeated high-force eccentric exercise: effects on muscle pain and damage. *Journal of Applied Physiology* **63,** 1381-1386

Schwane AJ, Johnson SR, Vandenakker CB & Armstrong RB (1983). Delayed onset muscle soreness and plasma CPK and LDH activities after downhill running. *Medicine and Science in Sports and Exercise* **15**, 51-56

Soares JMC, Duarte JA & Appell HJ (1992). Metabolic vs mechanic origin of muscle lesions induced by exercise. *International Journal of Sports Medicine* **13,** 84 (abstract)

Section IV

Muscle Performance: Mechanical Demand and Metabolic Supply

Human muscle fatigue in dynamic exercise

Anthony J. Sargeant and Anita Beelen

Department of Muscle and Exercise Physiology, Faculty of Human Movement Sciences, Vrije Universiteit, Meibergdreef 15, 1105 AZ Amsterdam, The Netherlands

Abstract   In humans, dynamic muscle funtion including fatigue has been studied less often than isometric function. There is however good evidence to show that the mode of exercise performed may determine both the type and the magnitude of the fatigue generated. Furthermore, since fatigue may affect both isometric force generation *and* the maximum velocity of shortening, characterisation of fatigue in terms of isometric force alone may grossly under-represent the true magnitude of the effect on power output. One reason for the relative neglect of dynamic function has been the technical difficulties associated with measuring human muscle power at known, or controlled, velocities which are realistic in terms of human locomotion. We describe the development of an isokinetic cycle ergometer which allows measurement of power output from the leg extensor muscles over a wide range of constant velocities. This enables the optimum velocity for power generation to be identified for this form of exercise. The application of this technique to study the effects of prior exercise and changes in muscle temperature are described together with observations on the pattern of muscle fibre type recruitment during dynamic exercise. The implications for human power output of having muscle composed of fibres with different contractile and metabolic properties are discussed in relation to maximum power output, sustained submaximal power, and mechanical efficiency.

Introduction - Measurement of human power output.

In human locomotion the ability to generate and sustain mechanical power output is of fundamental importance. In order to examine those factors which influence power output in the intact human we developed an isokinetic cycle ergometer (Sargeant, Hoinville and Young 1981; Sargeant and Dolan 1987; Beelen and Sargeant 1991, and 1992). The latest version has two operating modes and it can be instantly switched from one to the other (fig 1). In the lower configuration the ergometer is connected to a normal electrically braked cycle ergometer so that subjects can perform submaximal steady-state exercise. In the upper configuration the cycle is connected to an isokinetic control system. This consists of a large electric motor driving the cranks through a variable speed gearbox. Determinations of maximum power are made by switching on the isokinetic system at the chosen velocity and instructing the subject to make a maximum effort in an attempt to speed up the motor. Due to the characteristics of the motor-gear system this is not possible and pedalling rate is held constant. During the maximum effort the horizontal and vertical forces generated at the foot are continuously measured by means of strain gauges mounted in the pedals. Encoders record crank and pedal angles with respect to time enabling calculation of tangential (effective) force (fig 2). Integration of the force data with respect to velocity yields power output. In this review data for peak effective power will be presented, that is the instantaneous peak power generated during each crank revolution and tangential to the arc of the pedal axis trajectory - hence effective in terms of delivering power to the ergometer (fig 3). Generally this has been found to be representative of other measurements of power, such as the mean power calculated for the complete revolution (Sargeant, Hoinville and Young 1981; Beelen and Sargeant 1991, 1992).

    The strength of our approach is that we are measuring power generated by the main locomotory muscles at shortening velocities, that are realistic in terms of human locomotion. Technically the system has the merit that in this constrained form of exercise it is relatively easy to measure the forces generated on the pedals continuously and to control the crank velocity. The latter aspect is crucial since even though we are measuring power produced by the whole leg-hip complex, and not individual muscles, it is still necessary to take account of the 'global' power/velocity relationship of the active musculature. In figure 4 data is shown for 5 subjects in whom maximum peak power was measured in a series of experiments at different pedal rates ranging from 22 to 171 rev/min. The data is normalized to take account of the size of the active muscle mass and indicates an optimum pedalling rate for maximum power of between 110 to 120 rev/min (Sargeant et al 1981; Sargeant, Dolan and Young 1984; Sargeant and Dolan 1986).

An important issue that needs to be addressed is whether maximal activation of muscle can be achieved voluntarily in this repetitive dynamic exercise - we believe that the consensus of evidence indicates that it can. This is based on (a) studies where electrical stimulation has been superimposed on maximal voluntary dynamic contractions (Beelen, Sargeant, Jones, and de Ruiter 1993; James and Sacco 1992; Westing et al 1990); (b) EMG evidence which although indirect does not immediately suggest a failure of neural drive in fatigue (Greig, Hortobagyi and Sargeant 1985); (c) The fact that rather low maximal forces are generated in these fast dynamic contractions (< 50% of maximum isometric force) would seem to mitigate against the possibility of inhibitory reflexes influencing activation (Beelen and Sargeant 1991, 1992; Jones 1993).

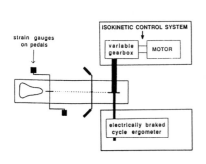

Figure 1. Diagram of the isokinetic cycle ergometer showing alternative coupling to an isokinetic device or to a conventional electrically braked cycle ergometer.

Figure 2. Sample of calculated tangential (effective) force generated on the pedal during 4 crank revolutions.

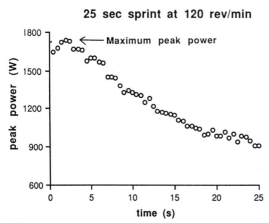

Figure 3. Calculated peak power for each revolution during a 25 s maximum effort performed at 120 rev/min.

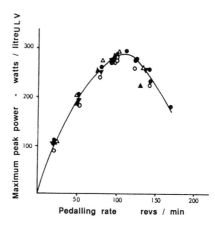

Figure 4. Relationship of maximum peak power to pedalling rate for 5 subjects. Power is standardised for the upper leg muscle volume (watts/litre$_{ULV}$). (Reprinted with permission from Sargeant et al 1981).

Human muscle fatigue in dynamic exercise

Fatiguing and potentiating effects of prior exercise

The data shown in Figure 4 is for maximum peak power of fresh muscle. In a subsequent study we examined the effect of performing a period of prior dynamic exercise on the maximum power output measured at optimal velocity. Firstly, we examined the effect of varying the duration of prior exercise performed at an intensity equivalent to 98% of maximum oxygen uptake ($\dot{V}O_{2max}$). Data for two subjects is shown in figure 5. As can be seen the maximum power is reduced as the duration of the prior exercise increases eventually stabilizing at about 70% of the control value between 3 and 6 mins. This response is suggestive of the obverse of the oxygen deficit seen at the start of exercise and it may similarly reflect the increased rate of energy turnover and the necessary utilization and depletion of anaerobic energy sources, notably phosphocreatine, at the start of exercise (Bangsbo et al 1989).

Using 6 minutes as the prior exercise duration we then examined the effect of different exercise intensities on power output. Figure 6 shows data for 5 subjects. It can be seen that low intensity prior exercise has a potentiating effect on power output.. At intensities above 60% $\dot{V}O_{2max}$ maximum peak power was increasingly reduced compared to control. The functional reduction in power appears to parallel the intensity dependent depletion of phosphocreatine (see e.g. Hultman et al 1967, Knuttgen and Saltin 1972).

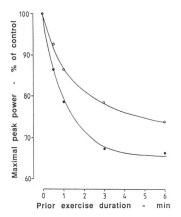
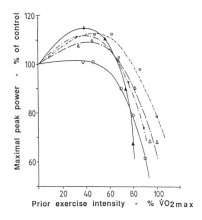

Figure 5. Maximum peak power (% control) determined in a series of experiments after different durations of prior exercise at 98% of $\dot{V}O_{2max}$. Individual data for 2 subjects (Sargeant and Dolan 1987).

Figure 6. Maximum peak power (% control) after 6 min of prior exercise performed at different intensities. Data for 5 subjects. (Sargeant and Dolan 1987).

In the last part of the study we examined the time course of recovery from this dynamically induced fatigue (figure 7). In a series of experiments we interposed a recovery period between a 6 min prior exercise bout performed at ~90% $\dot{V}O_{2max}$ and the determination of maximum power. In the absence of a recovery period the power output was reduced by 30 to 40%. Recovery of power was however shown to be a very rapid process with a half time of ~30 seconds so that maximum peak power had recovered within 1 minute of finishing the fatiguing prior exercise. After 6 min of recovery maximum power had significantly increased compared to control by ~+10%. The rapid recovery of power in these experiments follows a similar time course to that shown for the resynthesis of phosphocreatine following high intensity cycle ergometer exercise but contrasts markedly with the expected removal rate for lactate and the restoration of normal pH in the muscle, processes which may take 20 mins or longer (see e.g. respectively: Harris et al 1976; Sahlin et al 1976). These data obtained in recovery indicate that in *human muscle, in-vivo* , there can be an absence of fatigue even under acidotic conditions, supporting the suggestion that the link between hydrogen ion accumulation and fatigue is probably not a simple cause and effect, but rather indirect (Sahlin and Ren 1989). A point underlined by the experiments of Jones and his colleagues who demonstrated the occurrence of fatigue in human muscle even when glycolysis was absent and there was no rise in hydrogen ion concentration (Cady et al 1989).

In all three experiments reduced levels of phosphocreatine, consequent upon an energetic deficiency, would have lead to relatively large increases in ADP and Pi, both potential fatiguing agents, and severely limited the maximum rate of ADP rephosphorylation(Sahlin 1986).

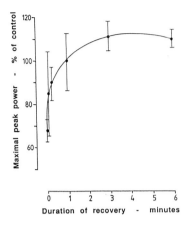

Figure 7. Recovery in maximum peak power after 6 min of prior exercise at ~90% $\dot{V}O_{2max}$. Mean ($\pm$ SD) data from 4 subjects (Sargeant and Dolan 1987).

Effect of changes in muscle temperature

The potentiating effects of prior exercise may partly be explained by an increase in muscle temperature (Sargeant 1987). Figure 8 summarizes the effect on the maximum peak power of manipulating muscle temperature by immersing the legs in water baths. Following 45 minutes standing in a water bath at 44°C muscle temperature was increased by 2.7°C compared to control and at optimal velocity this gave rise to an 11% increase in power. It can be seen that the magnitude of the effect is velocity dependent suggesting an increase in the maximum velocity of shortening (V_{max}). At the same time as increasing the maximum peak power there was an increase over the 20 second maximum effort in the rate of fatigue reflecting an increased rate of cross bridge cycling and utilization of high energy phosphate (figure 9).

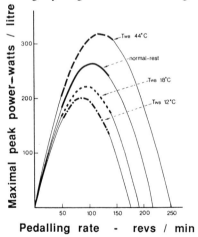

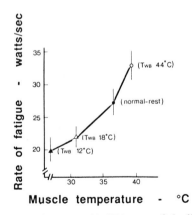

Figure 8. The relationship of maximum peak power to pedalling rate under normal rested conditions and following 45 min immersion in water baths at 44, 18, and 12°C. The thicker sections of the lines indicate the limits of the experimental data - the thinner sections the mathematical extrapolations (Sargeant 1987).

Figure 9. Mean ($\pm$ SD) rate of decline in peak power over 20 s maximum effort performed pedalling at 95 rev/min in relation to muscle temperature (measured at 3 cm depth in the mid anterior thigh). Water bath temperatures(T_{wb}) are given in brackets. (Reprinted with permission from Sargeant 1987)

Human muscle fatigue in dynamic exercise

Velocity dependent effect of fatigue

The effect of fatigue on dynamic function in the data presented so far was assessed in terms of human power output measured at optimal velocity (V_{opt}). Animal muscle experiments had demonstrated that fatigue resulted in changes not only in maximum isometric force, which was reduced by ~50%, but also in the force velocity characteristics, mainly due to a reduced maximum velocity of shortening (de Haan, Jones, and Sargeant 1989). Consequently characterisation of the fatigue only in terms of isometric force seriously under-represented the magnitude of the effect on maximum power (at V_{opt}) which was reduced by ~75%. Such an effect might have important implications for human locomotory performance where it could result in greater reductions in power at optimal and higher velocities compared to low velocities.

We examined this issue using our cycling model (Beelen and Sargeant 1991). In a series of experiments peak power was assessed at 5 different pedalling rates immediately following 6 minutes of exercise at 90% $\dot{V}O_{2\ max}$. Figure 10 shows the peak power for one subject at the lowest and highest pedalling rates studied. At 60 rev/min there was very little effect: In contrast, at 120 rev/min, there was a ~30% reduction in the maximum peak power. The data from 6 subjects show a clear velocity dependent effect on maximum peak power indicating a 'slowing' of the active muscles (figure 11). We interpreted these results as indicating a selective fatigue of faster fatigue sensitive muscle fibres which play a progressively greater role in power generation as velocity increases. This interpretation would also explain the apparent paradox shown in figure 10b of a faster rate of fatigue in the control compared to the fatigued state. The fatigue of peak power seen under control conditions is presumed to be due to a successive loss in the contribution from the most fatigue sensitive fibres - the effect of the prior exercise is that these fibres are already fatigued leaving a population of more fatigue resistant fibres.

In considering these data it should be remembered that the true magnitude of the velocity dependent effect of fatigue on power output may be somewhat obscured by an exercise induced increase in muscle temperature (+2.6°C). As already described this has an 'opposite' velocity dependent effect - increasing power output proportionately more at the higher velocities.

Finally it should be noted that the fatigue in these experiments was generated by dynamic exercise. When repetitive isometric contractions of the knee extensors were performed at 70% of MVC to produce a 30% fatigue of maximum isometric force there was a significant 7% reduction in power at 40 rev/min, but at 75 and 105 rev/min progressively smaller reductions of 4% and 2% were found which were not significant (Beelen and Sargeant 1989). This indicates that the type of exercise can determine not only the magnitude of the fatigue but also probably the site at which it occurs.

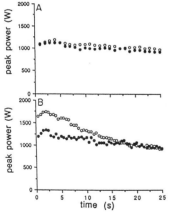
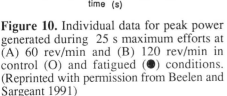
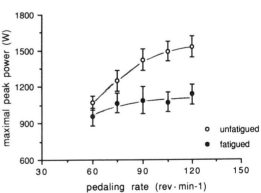

Figure 10. Individual data for peak power generated during 25 s maximum efforts at (A) 60 rev/min and (B) 120 rev/min in control (O) and fatigued (●) conditions. (Reprinted with permission from Beelen and Sargeant 1991)

Figure 11. Maximum peak power at 5 different pedalling rates in fatigued and unfatigued states. Mean (± SE) data for 6 subjects. (Beelen and Sargeant 1991)

Recruitment of different muscle fibre types in human dynamic exercise - the significance of contraction velocity

The suggestion of a selective effect of fatigue raises two important questions:

(i) *What is the potential contribution of different human fibre type populations to maximum power output at different contraction velocities?*

(ii) *How is that contribution moderated by the pattern of recruitment of different muscle fibre types during submaximal dynamic exercise?*

Some insight into the second question is gained from studies based on fibre type related patterns of glycogen depletion following dynamic exercise (see e.g. Gollnick et al 1972; Vollestad et al 1985, Vollestad and Blom 1985). On the assumption that in human muscle during relatively short duration exercise glycogen depletion in muscle fibres may be taken as indicative of contractile activity the results of these studies indicate a successive hierarchical recruitment of muscle fibre types. In the experiments of Vollestad et al cycle ergometer exercise was performed at a pedalling rate of 70 rev/min. The results indicate a successive recruitment of first type I fibres, next IIa, and finally type IIab and IIb fibres. At an exercise intensity of ~90% $\dot{V}O_{2\,max}$ virtually all fibres showed some degree of glycogen depletion even though the muscle only needed to generate ~50% of the maximum dynamic force available at that velocity of contraction (figure 12, Greig, Sargeant and Vollestad 1985). In a recent study in which subjects performed 12 minutes of exercise at 90% $\dot{V}O_{2\,max}$ we also found significant glycogen depletion in all fibre types (Beelen et al 1993). These findings imply a sub-maximal stimulation frequency, for some proportion of the fibres - presumably those at the top of the recruitment hierarchy. We would suggest that even this submaximal activation of the more sensitive fibre population may still be sufficient to cause fatigue.

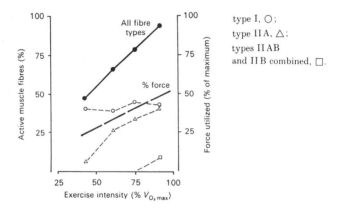

Figure 12. Proportion of available maximum force (i.e. as measured at the same pedalling rate - 70 rev/min) utilized, and muscle fibres active, in relation to exercise intensity. Values are also given for the component fibre type populations. (Reprinted with permission from Greig, Sargeant, and Vollestad 1985).

The experiments of Vollestad were conducted at a single pedalling rate. There are few data available on the effect of different movement frequencies on recruitment pattern. Gollnick et al (1972) did attempt to examine the question in a supplementary part to their main study but with the techniques available they were unable to identify any effect of different pedalling rates. Using a completely different approach we examined the functional consequences of prior exercise performed at different pedalling rates (Beelen and Sargeant 1992). When prior exercise performed at pedalling rates of 60 and 120 rev/min was matched for external power output (236W) there was evidence of a greater contribution at this submaximal exercise intensity from faster fibre populations at the faster pedalling rate .

Human muscle fatigue in dynamic exercise

The implications for human power output of fibre populations with different contractile properties

Maximum power output:

The first of the questions raised in the last section remains largely unanswered,

> *" What is the potential contribution of different human fibre type populations to maximum power output at different contraction velocities?"*

Faulkner et al (1981) measured the force velocity characteristics of bundles of human muscle fibres obtained at surgery. Taking account of the proportion of type I and II fibres present they suggested a ratio for the V_{max} of around 1:4. A similar ratio has more recently been proposed by Fitts et al (1989) and this ratio seems theoretically reasonable on dimensional grounds relative to other species (for a discussion of this point see e.g. Hill 1950, 1956, Rome et al 1990)

The implications for power output from human muscles which have fibre populations with different force velocity characteristics can be illustrated by reference to a model. For illustrative purposes the following assumptions and simplifications are made:

    (i)   That there are two discrete populations of muscle fibres (type I and II) with a 1:4 ratio for their maximum velocities of shortening.

    (ii) That the specific force of these two populations is such that when account is taken of their respective cross-sectional areas they each generate 50% of the whole muscle maximum isometric force.

    (iii) That the length tension relationships, relative to the whole muscle are the same for both fibre populations.

    (iv) That the a/Po constant which defines the curvature of the force velocity relationship is the same for both populations.

Of these **(i)** is a simplification to make the model manageable and comprehensible (see also the apparent plasticity of contractile properties of human muscle fibres as indicated by the training study of Fitts et al 1989; also training induced changes in myosin isoforms,Baumann et al 1987; Schantz and Dhoot 1987); **(ii)** is arbitary but not unreasonable for human mixed muscle; **(iii)** is a simplification, although on functional grounds one might expect differences related to the range over which task related recruitment of different fibre populations occurs.(see e.g. Herzog and ter Keurs 1987); **(iv)** is a simplification made in the absence of systematic data. It might be expected on the basis of animal muscle that the a/Po ratio is greater for the faster fibres thus making, if anything, the difference in power output even more dramatic (for a review see , Woledge Curtin and Homsher 1985, pp 47-56). The data of Fitts et al (1989) suggests differences in the a/Po constant between human type I and II fibres and also changes, especially in the type II fibres following intensive training.

The relative force and power velocity relationships for types I and II fibre populations in our hypothetical human muscle are shown in figure 13. If we assume a summation of power production from the two populations in the maximally activated whole muscle the combined power output will be as shown in figure 14. The great difficulty is to know how to relate the relative velocities of figures 13 and 14 to human locomotory movement. What we do know is that in cycling exercise the optimum pedalling rate for maximum power output is ~120 rev/min (figure 4). If it is assumed that this is the velocity at which the maximum power of the two populations combined is generated, then a pedalling rate of 60 rev/min approximates to the V_{opt} of the type I fibres. It also implies that the V_{max} of type I fibres will not be exceeded until a pedalling rate of ~ 165 rev/min is achieved and that the fastest fibres (type II) have an optimum velocity well in excess of that seen in normal locomotion. In general these implications from the model seem not unreasonable.

Sustained submaximum power output:

In locomotory function the ability to sustain submaximal levels of power is important. In figure 15 the x axis from figure 14 is expanded and submaximal power output levels approximating to .25 and 80% of the maximum power are indicated by dashed lines. At the 80% level of sustained power there is, by definition, a 20% reserve of the combined power generating capability when pedalling at 120 rev/min while at 60 rev/min there is no reserve. Similary at the 25% level there is a reserve of 75% at 120 rev/min but only 55% at 60 rev/min. On first consideration the greater reserves at the fast pedalling rate might suggest that this rate is preferable at *both* levels of power in terms of resisting fatigue and hence sustaining power output. In the case of the lower level of power output, however, this ignores the potential contribution to power output from the fatigue resistant type I fibres. In principle a power output of 25% of maximum could be achieved at 60 rev/min by recruiting *only* the type I fibres. At a pedalling rate of 120 rev/min, however, the same power output can only be attained if there is *minimally* a contribution of ~15% power from the faster type II fibre population - which ultimately includes fatigue sensitive fibres. Calculating for the model the *minimum possible* contribution from the type II fibres at different fractions of maximum power yields the data shown in figure 16.

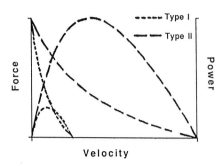

Figure 13. Force and power in relation to velocity for a slow (type I) and a fast (type II) population of fibres which have the same isometric force but V_{max} in the ratio of 1:4 (see the text for other qualifications).

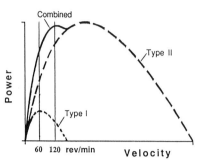

Figure 14. The component and combined power/velocity relationships for a whole muscle (modelled as if composed of two discrete populations of fibre types - see figure 13 and text). The velocity approximating to 120rev/min is derived from figure 5.

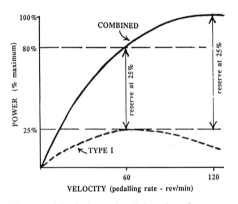

Figure 15. Submaximal levels of power (25 and 80% of maximum) in relation to the first part of the combined power/velocity relationship expanded from figure 14. The potential contribution of power from the type I fibre population is also given.

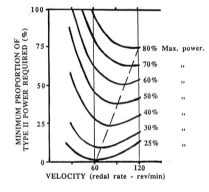

Figure 16. Relationship between the proportion of the type II power required and velocity at different fractions of maximum power - assuming that the type I population is contributing maximally (see text). The dashed line shows the progressive increase in the velocity at which the minimum contribution occurs. (based on figure 15)

This suggests that a low level of sustained power output (25% of maximum) the optimum pedalling rate to minimise the contribution required from type II fibres is 60 rev/min but at high levels of sustained power (80% of maximum) the optimum increases to 120 rev/min. It has already been pointed out that there is evidence for a significant element of rate coding superimposed on the hierarchical pattern of motor unit recruitment in this form of exercise (see also Ivy et al 1987). It should be emphasised therefore that this analysis is only describing the *minimum* contribution necessary from the *power generating capability* of the type II fibres - assuming an initial and full recruitment of the type I fibre population.

Human muscle fatigue in dynamic exercise

Interestingly, and despite all the assumptions and simplifications the model does seem to reflect real life. We recently had the opportunity to study a group of experienced competitive cyclists. They were asked to cycle at different constant speeds on their own bicycles and they were allowed to choose freely the gear at each speed studied (figure 17). It can be seen that as the exercise intensity increased so did their freely chosen pedal frequency - from ~60 rev/min at the lowest levels to ~110 at the highest (Sargeant and Beelen, unpublished observations.See also Pugh 1974).

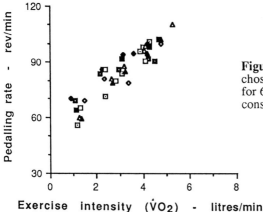

Figure 17. Relationship between the freely chosen pedalling rate and exercise intensity for 6 trained cyclists riding their bicycles at constant speed (20 to 47 km/hr).

Finally, it is worth considering the data derived from the world cycling record for distance achieved in one hour. Knowing the gear ratios the mean pedalling rate can be calculated. Over all the years analysed these world class athletes consistently chose a high pedalling rate of 104 (SD 2) rev/min in order to maintain a high sustained level of power output (Table 1).

YEAR	NAME	DISTANCE(km)	PEDAL RATE
1972	Merckx	49.431	104
1968	Ritter	48.653	105
1967	Bracke	48.093	106
1958	Riviere	47.347	105
1957	Riviere	46.923	106
1956	Baldini	46.394	104
1956	Anquetil	46.159	104
1942	Coppi	45.798	103
1937	Archambaud	45.767	104
1937	Slaats	45.485	104
1936	Richard	45.325	103
1935	Olmo	45.09	103
1933	Richard	44.777	102

Table 1. World records for 1 hour unpaced cycling (data courtesy of J Poulus).

Mechanical efficiency and pedalling rate

As pointed out previously (Sargeant 1988) the theoretical advantage described above of choosing fast pedalling rates at high levels of sustained submaximal power would be negated if there was a disproportionate increase in the energy cost for the same external power delivered - that is, mechanical efficiency decreased. Clearly however, at least in well trained cyclists, this is either (a)not the case, or (b)the advantage, in terms of fatigue resistance, outweighs the extra energy cost.

In fact as shown in figure 18, for a low level of external power the *total* energy cost of cycling at fast pedal rates (120 rev/min) is clearly higher than at slow rates (60 rev/min). This difference is however almost entirely the consequence of the (unmeasured) power that must be delivered in order to move the legs twice as often at the faster pedalling rate. The *delta* efficiency however is greater when cycling at 120 rev/min: that is the added energy cost for additional power output (calculated from the slope of the regressions VO₂/Power) is less at 120 than at 60 rev/min. Consequently there is a convergence of the VO₂/Power relationships at ~330 watts. Thus at the high levels of external power that can be delivered by well trained subjects in sustained 'steady state' aerobic exercise there appears to be no, or little, disadvantage in terms of energy cost in choosing fast pedalling rates (Sargeant 1988).

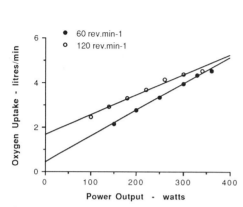

Figure 18. Relationship between oxygen uptake and external power output during cycle ergometer exercise pedalling at 60 and 120 rev/min. Individual data for a trained endurance athlete.

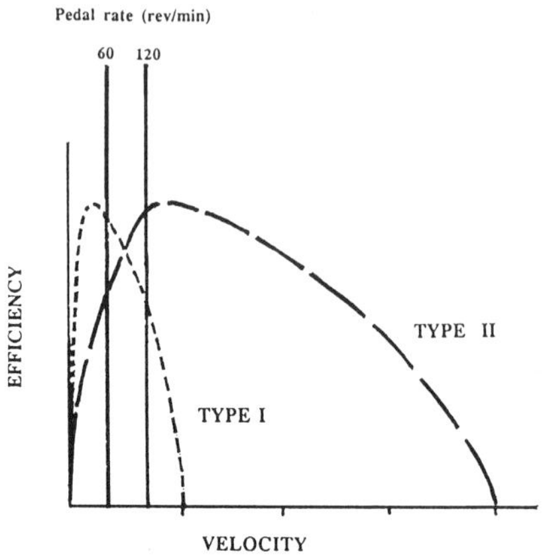

Figure 19. Schematic of the possible relationships between mechanical efficiency and velocity for the modelled fibre types. In the absence of systematic data no relative difference between the maximum efficiencies is given - each type is normalised to the same maximum. The velocity range equivalent to pedalling rates of 60 to 120 rev/min is derived from figure 14.

In the light of this observation it is of interest to consider how the mechanical efficiency of different human muscle fibre types may be influenced by the velocity of shortening. In order to examine the general principles type I and II fibres are again treated as if they were two discrete groups each of which is homogenous in it's properties (while recognising that the reality is somewhat different!) On the basis of animal muscle experiments it is usually proposed that maximum efficiency occurs at a velocity which is close to, but slightly below, the optimum for maximum power, e.g. 0.20 vs 0.30 V_{max} respectively (see e.g. Rome 1993). Using these values it can be speculated that the efficiency/velocity relationships for type I and II fibres might be of the general form shown in figure 19 (based on slow and fast animal muscle experiments; Goldspink 1978). By reference to the earlier discussion regarding the V_{opt} for maximum power in cycling it can be seen that the maximum efficiency for the type I fibres would occur at ~ 35 rev/min and for type II fibres at ~130 rev/min. In high intensity exercise, where both fibre types make a substantial contribution to power output, pedalling rate may have little effect since there may be reciprocal changes in the efficiency of the two fibre types. But it should be remembered that this conclusion is based on a simplified model. As with other contractile properties the efficiency/velocity relationship can be expected to be rather 'plastic' and with reference to the earlier discussion may be influenced by, e.g. the a/Po constant (Woledge 1968). In these circumstances it will be necessary to carefully specify the training status, fibre composition, and exercise intensity/recruitment pattern, if any meaningful conclusions regarding the efficiency/velocity relationship of human muscle fibre types are to be drawn from whole body exercise.

Human muscle fatigue in dynamic exercise

References

Bangsbo, J., Gollnick, P.D., Graham, T.E., Juel, C., Kiens, B., Mizuno, M. & Saltin, B. (1990). Anaerobic energy production and O_2 deficit-debt relationship during exhaustive exercise in man. *Journal of Physiology* **422**, 539-559.

Baumann, H., Jaggi, M., Soland, F., Howald, H. & Schaub, M.C. (1987). Exercise training induces transitions of myosin isoform subunits within histochemically typed human muscle fibers. *Pflügers Archiv.European Journal of Physiology* **409**, 349-360.

Beelen, A. & Sargeant, A.J. (1989). Effect of fatigue on maximum short term power output at different contraction velocities in humans. *Journal of Physiology* **409,** 22P.

Beelen, A. & Sargeant, A.J. (1991). Effect of fatigue on maximal power output at different contraction velocities in humans. *Journal of Applied Physiology* **71**, (6), 2332-2337.

Beelen, A. & Sargeant, A.J. (1992). Effect of prior exercise at different pedal frequencies on maximal power in humans. *European Journal of Applied Physiology*. (In press).

Beelen, A., Sargeant, A.J., Jones, D.A.& de Ruiter, C.J. (1993). Fatigue and recovery of voluntary and electrically elicited dynamic force in humans. In: *Neuromuscular Fatigue*. Eds., Sargeant, A.J., and Kernell, D. Academy Series. Royal Netherlands Academy of Arts and Sciences - Elsevier, Amsterdam.

Beelen, A., Sargeant, A.J., Lind, A., de Haan, A. Kernell, D. & van Mechelen, W. (1993). Effect of contraction velocity on the pattern of glycogen depletion in human muscle fibre types. In: *Neuromuscular Fatigue*. Eds., Sargeant, A.J., and Kernell, D. Academy Series. Royal Netherlands Academy of Arts and Sciences - Elsevier, Amsterdam.

Cady, E.B., Jones, D.A., Lynn, J. & Newham, D.J. (1989). Changes in force and intracellular metabolites during fatigue of human skeletal muscle. *Journal of Physiology* **418**, 311-325.

de Haan, A., Jones, D.A. & Sargeant, A.J. (1989). Changes in power output, velocity of shortening and relaxation rate during fatigue of rat medial gastrocnemius muscle. *Pflügers Archiv. European Journal of Physiology* **413**, 422-428.

Faulkner, J.A., Jones, D.A., Round, J.M. & Edwards, R.H.T. (1980). Dynamics of energetic processes in human muscle. *Exercise Bioenergetics and Gas Exchange*, P. Cerretelli & B.J. Whipp (Eds.), Elsevier / North-Holland Biomedical Press.

Fitts, R.H., Costill, D.L. & Gardetto, P.R. (1989). Effect of swim training on human muscle fiber function. *Journal of Applied Physiology* 66 (1), 465-475.

Goldspink, G. (1978). Energy turnover during contraction of different types of muscle. *Biomechanics VI-A*, E. Asmussen and K. Jørgensen (Eds.). Baltimore University Park Press, pp. 27-39.

Greig, C.A., Sargeant, A.J. & Vollestad, N.K. (1985). Muscle force and fibre recruitment during dynamic exercise in man. *Journal of Physiology* **371**, 176P.

Greig, C.A., Hortobagyi, T. & Sargeant, A.J. (1985). Quadriceps surface e.m.g., and fatigue during maximal dynamic exercise in man. *Journal of Physiology* 369, 180P.

Harris, R.C., Edwards, R.H.T., Hultman, E. & Nordesjö, L-O. (1976). Phosphagen and lactate contents of m. quadriceps femoris of man after exercise. *Journal of Physiology* **367**: 137-142.

Herzog, W. & ter Keurs, H.E.D.J. (1988). Force-length relation of in-vivo human rectus femoris muscles. *Pflügers Archiv. European Journal of Physiology* **411**, 642-647.

Hill, A.V. (1950). The dimensions of animal and their muscular dynamics. *Proceedings Royal Institute of Great Britain* **34**, 450-473.

Hill, A.V. (1956). The design of muscles. *British Medical Bulletin* **12**, 165-166.

Hultman, E., Bergström, J. & McLennan-Anderson, N. (1967). Breakdown and resynthesis of PC and ATP in connection with muscular work in man. *Scandinavian Journal of Clinical Laboratory Investigations* **19**, 56-66.

Ivy, J.L., Chi, M-Y., Hintz, C.S., Sherman, W.M., Hellendall, R.P. & Lowry, O.H. (1987). Progressive metabolic changes in individual human muscle fibers with increasing work rates. *American Journal of Physiology* **252**, C630-C639.

James, C. & Sacco (1992). Central and peripheral fatigue during sustained dynamic exercise. *Journal of Physiology*. In Press.

Jones, D.A. (1993). How far can experiments in the laboratory explain the fatigue of athletes in the field. In: *Neuromuscular Fatigue*. Eds., Sargeant, A.J., and Kernell, D. Academy Series. Royal Netherlands Academy of Arts and Sciences - Elsevier, Amsterdam.

Knuttgen, K.G. & Saltin, B. (1972). Muscle metabolites and O_2 uptake in short-term submaximal exercise in man. *Journal of Applied Physiology* **32**, 690-694.

Pugh, L.G.C.E. (1974). The relation of oxygen intake and speed in competition cycling and comparative observations on the bicycle ergometer. *Journal of Physiology* **241**, 795-808.

Rome, L.C., Sosnicki, A.A. & Goble, D.O. (1990). Maximum velocity of shortening of three fibre types from horse soleus muscle: implications for scaling with body size. *Journal of Physiology* **431**, 173-185.

Rome, L. (1993). The design of the muscular system. In: *Neuromuscular Fatigue*. Eds., Sargeant, A.J., and Kernell, D. Academy Series. Royal Netherlands Academy of Arts and Sciences - Elsevier, Amsterdam.

Sahlin, K. (1986). Metabolic changes limiting muscle performance. In: Saltin B. (Eds.) Biochemistry of Exercise VI p.p. 323-343. Human Kinetics, Champaign Ill.

Sahlin, K. & Ren, J.M. (1989). Relationship of contraction capacity to metabolic changes during recovery from a fatiguing contraction. *Journal of Applied Physiology* **67**, 648-654.

Sahlin, K., Harris, R.C., Nyland, B. & Hultman, E. (1976). Lactate content and pH in muscle samples obtained after dynamic exercise. *Pflügers Archiv. European Journal of Physiology* **367**, 143-149.

Sargeant, A.J. (1987). Effect of muscle temperature on leg extension force and short-term power output in humans. *European Journal of Applied Physiology* **56**, 693-698.

Sargeant, A.J. (1988). Optimum cycle frequencies in human movement. *Journal of Physiology* **406**, 49P.

Sargeant, A.J. & Dolan, P. (1986). Optimal velocity of muscle contraction for short-term (anaerobic) power output in children and adults. (pp 39-42) In: *Children and Exercise XII*, eds. Rutenfranz, J., Mocellin, R. and Klimt, F. Human Kinetics Publishers. Champaign, Ill.

Sargeant, A.J. & Dolan, P. (1987). Effect of prior exercise on maximal short-term power output in man. *Journal of Applied Physiology* **63**, 1475-1482.

Sargeant, A.J., Dolan, P. & Young, A. (1984). Optimal velocity for maximal short-term anaerobic power output in cycling. *International Journal of Sports Medicine* **5**, 124-125.

Sargeant, A.J., Hoinville, E. & Young, A. (1981). Maximum leg force and power output during short-term dynamic exercise. *Journal of Applied Physiology* **51** (5), 1175-1182.

Schantz, P.G. & Dhoot, G.K. (1987). Coexistence of slow and fast isoforms of contractile and regulatory proteins in human skeletal muscle fibers induced by endurance training. *Acta Physiologica Scandinavica* **131**, 147-154.

Vøllestad, N.K. & Blom, P.C.S. (1985). Effect of varying exercise intensity on glycogen depletion in human muscle fibers. *Acta Physiologica Scandinavica* **125**, 395-405.

Vøllestad, N.K., Vaage, O. & Hermansen, L. (1984). Muscle glycogen depletion patterns in type I and subgroups of type II fibres during prolonged severe exercise in man. *Acta Physiologica Scandinavica* **122**, 433-441.

Westing, S.H., Seger, J.Y. & Thorstensson, A. (1990). Effects of electrical stimulation on eccentric torque-velocity relationships during knee extension in man. *Acta Physiologica Scandinavica* **140**, 17-22.

Woledge, R.C. (1968). The energetics of tortoise muscle. *Journal of Physiology* **197**, 685-707.

Woledge, R.C., Curtin, N.A. & Homsher, E. (1985). Energetic aspects of muscle contraction. *Monographs of the Physiological Society* No. **41**. Academic Press London.

Discussion

We had hypothesised that there would be a relatively greater proportional contribution to the mechanical power output of the whole muscle from type II muscle fibres at the higher pedalling rate. Further we expected that this would be reflected in greater energy turnover and glycogenolysis in those fibres. Insofar as there was a significant greater glycogen depletion in type IIB fibres after exercise at 120 rev/min compared with exercise at 60 rev/min our expectations were confirmed. There was also however a tendency for an increased depletion in type I and IIA fibres and at first sight this is somewhat surprising.

Clearly however these results do not support the conclusion, based on EMG data, of Citterio and Agostoni (1984) that there is a derecruitment of type I fibres at fast pedalling rates.

It must be realised that in comparing exercise performed at 60 with exercise performed at 120 rev/min not only contraction velocity is different but also the number of contractions. Since during exercise at 120 rev/min twice as many contractions are performed than during exercise at 60 rev/min, the (mechanical) start-up costs will be twice that during exercise at 60 rev/min. It does seem possible that although type I fibres are recruited during exercise at 120 rev/min they are operating on the descending arm of a mechanical efficiency/velocity relationship (see Rome 1993; and Sargeant and Beelen 1993). The consequence would be that proportionately more power would need to be generated by the type II fibre populations and together with the increased start-up costs this may lead to an increased glycogenolysis in both type I and type II fibres.

References

Beelen, A., and Sargeant, A.J. (1991). Effect of prior exercise at two different shortening velocities in humans. *Journal of Applied Physiology: Respiratory, Environmental, and Exercise Physiology* **71**, 2332-2337.

Beelen, A., and Sargeant, A.J. (1992). Effect of prior exercise at different pedal frequencies on maximal power in humans. *European Journal of Applied Physiology (in press)*

Citterio, G., and Agostoni, E.(1984). Selective activation of quadriceps muscle fibers according to bicycling rate. *Journal of Applied Physiology: Respiratory, Environmental, and Exercise Physiology* **57**, 371-379.

Gollnick, P.D., Piehl, K., Saltin, B. (1974). Selective glycogen depletion pattern in human muscle fibres after exercise of varying intensity and at varying pedalling rates. *Journal of Physiology London)* **241**, 45-57.

Kleinbaum, D.G., Kupper L.L., and Muller, K.E. (1988). *Applied regression analysis and other multi-variable methods.* (p.p. 298-299) Second Edition, PWS-KENT Publishers, Boston.

Rome, L. (1993). The design of the muscular system. In: *Neuromuscular Fatigue.* Eds.: Sargeant, A.J., and Kernell, D. Academy Series. Royal Netherlands Academy of Arts and Sciences and Sciences-Elsevier, Amsterdam.

Sargeant, A.J., Hoinville, E., and Young, A. (1981). Maximum leg force and power output during short term dynamic exercise. *Journal of Applied Physiology: Respiratory, Environmental, and Exercise Physiology* **50**, 1175-1182.

Sargeant, A.J. (1988). Optimum cycle frequencies in human movement. *Journal of Physiology* **406**, 49P.

Sargeant, A.J., and Beelen, A. (1993). Human muscle fatigue in dynamic exercise. In: *Neuromuscular Fatigue.* Eds.: Sargeant, A.J., and Kernell, D. Academy Series. Royal Netherlands Academy of Arts and Sciences and Sciences-Elsevier, Amsterdam.

Vøllestad, N.K., Vaage, O., and Hermansen, L. (1984). Muscle glycogen depletion patterns in type I and subgroups of type II fibres during prolonged severe exercise in man. *Acta Physiologica Scandinavica* **122**, 433-441.

Gradual increase in metabolic rate during repeated isometric contractions

N.K. Vøllestad & E. Saugen

Dep. of Physiology, National Institute of Occupational Health, Box 8149 Dep, N-0033 OSLO, Norway

It is generally agreed that fatigue during a sustained contraction is associated with a decreased ATP:force ratio (Wilkie 1986). In prolonged dynamic exercise, on the other hand, oxygen uptake remains almost constant (Åstrand & Rodahl 1986) and hence there is little evidence that the energy cost of contraction decreases. We have recently shown that leg oxygen uptake increases gradually by about 100 % from the first minutes of exercise till exhaustion during repeated 30 % MVC contractions (Vøllestad *et al.* 1990). This observation suggests a temporal increase in the rate of ATP utilization or a less efficient ATP synthesis in the mitochondria.

In an attempt to investigate these mechanisms more closely, we conducted a new series of similar experiments. We wanted to examine to what extent recruitment of unfatigued type II fibres (presumably less efficient) contributes to the increased energy turnover. Test contractions at either 30 % MVC or 50 % MVC were generated repeatedly during the fatiguing exercise. It was assumed that only a small fraction of type II fibres were active during 30 % MVC in the initial part of the exercise. At later stages these fibres became more active due to fatigue in the fibres activated from start. In the 50 % MVC contractions, however, it is expected that most of the type II fibres are active even in the control, unfatigued contractions. Hence, if recruitment of less efficient type II fibres plays an important role for the increased energy turnover, the 30 % MVC contractions should show a larger response.

Methods

Six subjects carried out isometric knee-extensor contractions with both legs simultaneously. The target force was 30 % MVC and these contractions were held for 6 s with 4 s rest between. Before start, unfatigued control contractions were carried out at 30 % and 50 % MVC, held for 15 s or 10 s, respectively. During the fatiguing exercise, test contractions (alternating 30 % and 50 % MVC) were carried out every third minute.

The rate of temperature rise (dT/dt) was measured from 2-4 thermocouples inserted into the vastus lateralis muscle. Temperature rose linearly during contraction (Fig. 1). To avoid disturbance from the movement artifacts at onset and release of contraction, dT/dt was determined by linear regression analysis from 2 s after onset of contraction to 1 s before release.

Results

In control contractions dT/dt was 5.3 and 10.1 mK/s during 30 % and 50 % MVC, respectively. After onset of the repeated 30 % MVC contractions (6 s on and 4 s off) dT/dt rose gradually for both test contraction levels. After 30 min dT/dt was 7.6 mK/s for the 30 % and 15 mK/s for the 50 % MVC contractions. Hence, the relative changes were 40 and 48 %. Intramuscular temperature showed a quite different temporal relationship, with a fast initial increase of about 3°C, but remained stable after about 20 min.

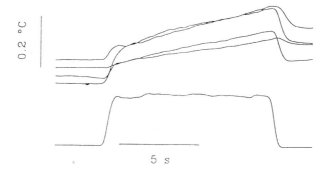

0.2 °C

5 s

Figure 1. Four simultaneous registrations of temperature rise in the vastus lateralis muscle during a 50 % MVC contraction. Lower tracing shows force. The data are low- pass filtered (3 Hz).

Discussion

Since the rise in heat production was comparable to the increase in leg oxygen uptake previously reported (Vøllestad *et al.* 1990), the increased energy turnover during repeated isometric contractions is localized to the muscle itself. The relative changes in heat production were less for the 30 % MVC contractions as compared with the 50 % MVC contractions. Hence, recruitment of less energy efficient type II fibres cannot be the sole explanation for the increased energy turnover. This conclusion is in agreement with earlier observations showing a sudden 75% decline in CrP at exhaustion, indicating that in most of the fibres (including type I fibres) glycolysis and oxidative phosphorylation became insufficient to meet the energy demand of the cells (Vøllestad *et al.* 1988). We therefore conclude the increased energy turnover occured at the cellular level.

The mechanisms behind this change could be either a less efficient mitochondrial resynthesis of ATP (reduced P:O ratio) or a less efficient ATP utilization (less force generated per ATP utilized). Since the test contractions lasted 15 s or 10 s, their energy demand exceeded the maximum amount of stored oxygen by a factor of 2. Hence, it may be expected a switch from anaerobic metabolism in the early part of contraction to anaerobic processes in the final stages. Temperature rose linearly during the entire test contractions throughout the exercise period. Hence, the increased energy consumption was probably attributable to an increased rate of ATP utilization per force rather than a less efficient ATP synthesis.

References

Åstrand PO & Rodahl K (1986). *Textbook of Work Physiology. Physiological Bases of Exercise*. McGraw-Hill Book Company. New York. USA.

Vøllestad NK, Sejersted OM, Bahr R, Woods JJ & Bigland-Ritchie B (1988). Motor drive and metabolic responses during repeated submaximal contractions in man. *Journal of Applied Physiology* **64**, 1421-1427.

Vøllestad NK, Wesche J & Sejersted OM (1990). Gradual increase in leg oxygen uptake during repeated submaximal contractions in humans. *Journal of Applied Physiology* **68**, 1150-1156.

Wilkie DR (1986). Muscular fatigue: effects of hydrogen ions and inorganic phosphate. *Federation Proceedings* **45**, 2921-2923.

Fatigue of intermittently stimulated quadriceps during imposed cyclical lower leg movements

Henry M. Franken, Peter H. Veltink and Herman B.K. Boom

University of Twente, Department of Electrical Engineering, The Netherlands

Introduction

A major issue in the control of functional electrical stimulation (FES) of paralysed muscles is the decay of muscle force as a result of fatigue under sustained (continuous and intermittent) stimulation (Andrews et al 1989, Boom et al 1992, Levy et al 1990, Mulder et al submitted). Stimulated paralyzed human quadriceps fatigue under isometric condition can be described by an exponential decay (Boom et al 1992, Levy et al 1990, Mulder et al submitted). In this study the torque of intermittently stimulated paralysed human knee extensors during (isokinetic) cyclical lower leg movements has been investigated.

Methods

A protocol was designed to compare overall loss of tetanic torque at the knee joint during sustained intermittent stimulation at different isokinetic velocities. The angle and velocity ranges were limited by the anatomical restrictions of the lower leg, the restrictions imposed by the experimental set-up (a KINCOM 125ES (Kinetic Communicator Exercise System) dynamometer bench) and the desire to maintain a constant cycle time, comparable to a walking cycle. The experimental set-up is shown in figure 1. The influence of duty cycle and stimulation frequency, at isokinetic joint movement, was also investigated. Identification trials, determining the torque-angle (isometric) and torque-angular velocity (isokinetic, measured at 40 deg. of knee flexion) relations, were performed. Pulsewidth and amplitude were set to obtain maximal recruitment. The interpulse intervals (IPI) used were 20 and 40 msec, both ensuring a fused contraction. Force, angular position, and velocity were sampled at 100 Hz. These signals and stimulus data were stored on disk for off-line analysis.

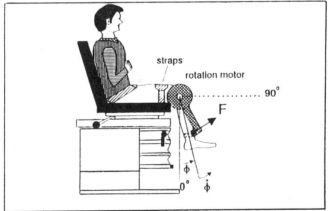

Figure 1. Schematic of experimental set-up. The angular position and velocity, measured at the motor axis, are defined positive in extension motion with zero as indicated. The patient is strapped at the hip and above the knee to measure knee torque (at the tibia) only and to ensure static position of the body.

The subjects who participated in this study were complete T5-T6 level spinal cord injured patients. All had normal excitable quadriceps muscle and had been enrolled in the FES training program of the rehabilitation center *'t Roessingh* (Enschede, The Netherlands).

Results

From the resulting torque, obtained by subtracting the averaged passive torque from the measured torque at the knee, the maximum and torque-time integral (TTI) per swing were calculated. The TTI was obtained by summating over a constant time period of the swing where the contraction takes place, including activation and relaxation phases, with constant velocity. The typical exponential decay of isometric quadriceps torque, reaching asymptotic values (Boom et al 1992, Levy et al 1990, Mulder et al submitted), resembles the overall loss of tetanic torque and TTI during sustained intermittent stimulation at isokinetic condition as found in this study. Additionally, the results indicate a significant dependence of the rate and magnitude of decay on the contraction velocity, which has not been reported before. Higher velocities result in a larger and faster decay of maximal torque and TTI. Also, the rate and magnitude of fatigue for concentric contractions appears to be directly related to duty cycle and 1/IPI.

Electrically stimulated muscle is a nonlinear dynamic system, exhibiting nonlinear dependence on position and velocity, which make it extremely difficult to control. Our identification results resemble the output of muscle model structures reported in animal experiments. The typical Gaussian-type dependence of the generated torque on the angle was also found. Hill's equation, favoured by many researchers for curve-fitting the torque-velocity relation for concentric contractions, is also representative for our results.

Discussion

The dependence of the fatigue curve of transcutaneously stimulated human quadriceps on the isokinetic knee joint velocity and the applied stimulation parameters (duty cycle, IPI) is an important factor in the design of optimal control systems for FES which pursue minimization of muscle fatigue. Basically, the results given above indicate that within the (lower) boundary conditions for a given task (ontime/IPI), which is equal to the number of pulses given, should be minimized to postpone fatigue. The results may contribute to the derivation of an optimization criterion, describing muscle fatigue as a function of both joint movement and stimulation parameters.

References

Andrews BJ, Barnett RW, Phillips GF and Kirkwood CA: Rule-based control of a hybrid FES orthosis for assisting paraplegic locomotion. *Automedica* 11:175-199, 1989.

Boom HBK, Mulder AJ and Veltink PH: Fatigue during finite state control during neuromuscular stimulation, *Progress in Brain Research,* in press, 1992.

Levy M, Mizrahi J and Susak Z: Recruitment, force and fatigue characteristics of quadriceps muscles of paraplegics isometrically activated by surface functional electrical stimulation, *J. Biomed. Eng.* 12:150-156, 1990.

Mulder AJ, Scheerder COS, Veltink PH, Boom HBK and Zilvold G: Muscle fatigue during continuous and intermittent transcutaneous stimulation of human quadriceps, Submitted to *IEEE Trans Biomed. Eng.*

How far can experiments in the laboratory explain the fatigue of athletes in the field?

D.A. Jones

Department of Physiology, University College London, Gower Street, London WC1E 6BT.

Abstract Much of the work on muscle fatigue in the past has concentrated on sustained isometric contractions yet in sporting events fatigue is most apparent as a result of high intensity shortening contractions. Although the rate of fatigue during dynamic exercise is greater than during isometric contractions there is little evidence to suggest that the former are more susceptible to central fatigue. Measurements of intracellular metabolites show that the ATP turnover of a shortening contraction is approximately twice that of an isometric contraction. In addition, the ability to sustain force whilst shortening is also more affected by the metabolic changes occurring during fatigue than is the ability to generate isometric force. The loss of power is associated with a slowing of the fatigued muscle.

Work in the last 40 years has highlighted a number of aspects of muscle function which may be at risk during muscle fatigue. These aspects include the question of central as opposed to peripheral fatigue, the neuromuscular junction, the surface membrane, excitation/contraction coupling and the role of muscle metabolites in modulating force. While significant progress has been made in understanding the changes which occur during isometric contractions there is still a gap in our understanding of the causes of fatigue during everyday and sporting activities.

Changes in power output during high intensity exercise

During a sprint, sustained high power output is required first to accelerate the body and then to maintain the running speed by overcoming air resistance and other frictional losses. The changes in maximum power output during a sprint are illustrated in Fig 1a, which shows that, after a peak in the first few seconds, power falls rapidly so that by 30s it is reduced to 50 or 60% of the maximum value. Earlier work by Sargeant *et al* (1981) using an isokinetic bicycle showed a similar rapid loss of power during all-out exercise.

The loss of power is remarkable when compared to the fatigue seen during sustained isometric contractions (Fig 1b). During the isometric contraction there was a modest loss of force so that by 30s only about 20% of the initial force had been lost. Similar rates of force loss are seen in other human muscles performing sustained isometric contractions.

The difference between the rates of fatigue illustrated in Figs 1a and 1b is all the more dramatic in view of the fact that the isometric contraction was made under ischaemic conditions while, during the dynamic exercise, the muscles were contracting intermittently for relatively short periods during each stride so there was the opportunity for recovery as the blood returned.

I will consider three reasons for the difference in time course. The first possibility is that a subject may find the rapid, intermittent dynamic movements involved in running more difficult to sustain than a simple isometric contraction, that is, the extent of "central" fatigue may be greater.

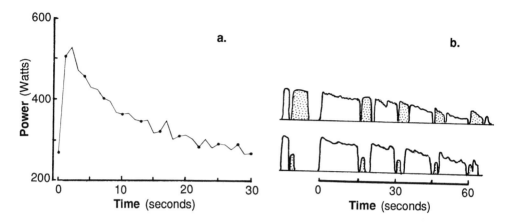

Figure 1. a. Power output of well trained athletes sprinting on a free running treadmill (Cheetham *et al*, 1986). **b.** Comparison of the force obtained by electrical stimulation with voluntary force during a sustained maximum voluntary contraction of the quadriceps. Above, femoral nerve stimulation, below, percutaneous stimulation; stimulated contractions are shaded (Bigland-Ritchie *et al*, 1978).

The second possibility is that dynamic exercise is more metabolically demanding and, whatever the link between metabolic depletion and fatigue, dynamic contractions will invoke this process sooner or to a greater extent than during an isometric contraction. The third possibility is that the ability of a muscle to generate force during shortening contractions may be more sensitive to the biochemical changes occurring during exercise than is the ability to sustain isometric force. Preliminary data will be presented which address each of these topics.

Central fatigue during dynamic exercise

Merton (1954) was the first to use electrical stimulation to study the question of central activation during fatiguing activity and concluded that full activation could be maintained during a maximum voluntary contraction sustained for three minutes. This has been confirmed with well motivated and experienced subjects making contractions of the adductor pollicis (Bigland-Ritchie *et al*, 1983) and, with some reservations, for contractions of the quadriceps lasting one minute (Fig 1b). During rapid dynamic exercise, contractions are brief and there is limited feedback about the performance of any one muscle and consequently any hesitation or reluctance to use a fatigued muscle might be expected to be more apparent during this form of exercise.

In theory it should be possible to use the technique of superimposing electrical stimulation to monitor the development of central fatigue during dynamic exercise. In practice it is difficult to stimulate sufficiently to record an unequivocal increase in force when the voluntary force is varying as a result of a change in joint angle, length of the muscle and the normal pattern of rhythmic activation. Nevertheless the method has been used by Newham *et al* (1991) who found that with fatigued muscle at low velocities of knee extension (20°/s) the degree of central inhibition was similar to that seen with isometric contractions but at higher speeds (150°/s) there was no detectable inhibition. James & Sacco (1992) found little or no evidence of central fatigue using femoral nerve stimulation during contractions at 90°/s.

Despite the experimental evidence, there may be lingering doubts as to whether the results illustrated in Fig 1a and 1b represent differences in the behaviour of the muscle rather than of the mind. The two types of activity can be compared using electrically stimulated isometric and dynamic exercise. Tetanic isometric contractions of the adductor pollicis were recorded before and after a period of exercise under ischaemic conditions. In one case the fatiguing exercise was a 10s isometric tetanus while, in the other, the muscle was stimulated and allowed to shorten against a load. The shortening contraction lasted 0.1s and was repeated every second for 100 seconds so that the total time of stimulation was the same in the two types of activity. The isometric fatiguing protocol resulted in only minor changes in force (10% loss) and relaxation rate of the test tetani but the dynamic fatiguing protocol had major effects with 50% force loss and pronounced slowing of relaxation. This observation confirms that there are major differences in the muscular response to isometric and dynamic exercise.

Energy demands of different forms of exercise

We have measured the phosphorus metabolites of the adductor pollicis by magnetic resonance spectroscopy (MRS). Spectra were collected under ischaemic conditions before and after maximal activity with the muscles stimulated either isometrically for 5 seconds at 50Hz or for 0.1s once every second for 50 seconds with the muscle free to shorten against a load equal to about 30% of the isometric force. Table 1 shows the metabolite values for the resting muscle and the values after the periods of isometric or dynamic exercise. During the dynamic exercise more phosphocreatine was broken down and an even greater quantity of lactate was formed when compared to the isometric contraction. The metabolic cost of the dynamic contraction (9.3 mM ATP/s) was approximately twice that of the isometric contraction (4.7 mM ATP/s). The differences were not a consequence of the longer overall duration of the dynamic exercise as the resting metabolic rate is about 1000 times less than the active turnover whether measured in fresh muscle or after a period of activity.

	Pi	PCr	ATP	pH	ΔLactate
Rest	8.2±0.3	30.0±0.6	8.2±1.1	7.18±0.04	
Isometric	19.9±1.0	18.3±0.4	7.9±0.4	7.06±0.01	7.5
Dynamic	25.1±1.0	11.6±0.9	7.5±0.4	6.78±0.04	18.3

Table 1. Metabolite contents of human adductor pollicis at rest and following activity. ^{31}P-MRS spectra were collected using methods very similar to those described by Cady *et al* (1989a). Measurements were made before and after either an isometric tetanus or a similar period of dynamic exercise. Values are given as mmoles per litre intracellular water and are the mean ± SEM of 20 measurements on resting muscles and 10 following each form of exercise, made on the same five subjects.

Differential effects of fatigue on isometric and shortening contractions

A feature of acutely fatigued muscle is slow relaxation from an isometric tetanus (Fig 2a).

It has been argued that there may be some benefits to be gained from slow relaxation for the maintenance of isometric force in that, as the fusion frequency decreases, the same force can be generated with a lower motoneurone firing frequency. It has also been pointed out that, if the slowing involves a reduction in cross bridge cycling, then while isometric force may be preserved, force generated during shortening would be reduced (Jones & Bigland-Ritchie, 1986). It is important to know the extent to which these possible differential effects of fatigue on isometric force and power output may affect human muscle.

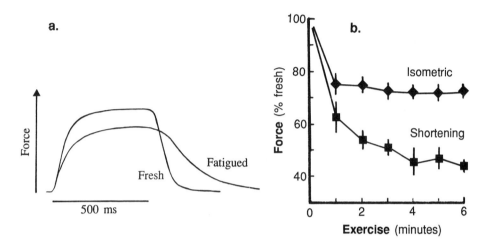

Figure 2. a. Relaxation of force at the end of a brief tetanus of fresh muscle and after 30s fatiguing contraction; note the increased half time of relaxation. First dorsal interosseous of the human hand (Cady *et al*, 1989b). **b.** The force obtained by electrical stimulation of the quadriceps, first held isometric and then allowed to shorten isokinetically. One subject exercised for 6 minutes and was tested every minute (mean $\pm$ SEM of 5 runs).

Fig 2b shows results from a subject exercising the quadriceps muscles isokinetically at 90°/s. Every minute the muscle was stimulated via the femoral nerve to produce a maximal isometric tetanus and the leg was then released into a shortening contraction. The isometric force and the dynamic force (measured at 60° knee flexion) both decreased with time but the extent of force loss for the shortening contraction (about 50%) was roughly twice the loss of isometric force (James & Jones, 1990), showing there is a difference in the ability of fatigued muscle to generate power and isometric force.

This phenomenon was examined in more detail using the human adductor pollicis. The stimulated muscle was allowed to shorten against loads ranging from about 0.05 to 0.6 Po. A length transducer attached to the thumb was used to measure the velocity of shortening and force-velocity curves were obtained for the fresh muscle. A cuff was inflated around the arm and the muscle fatigued and tested using a sequence of 1s tetani (50Hz) which consisted of five isometric contractions followed by four shortening contractions against different loads. This sequence was repeated four times, recording the force and relaxation rate of the last isometric tetanus in each sequence together with the speed of the isotonic shortening contractions.

Fig 3a shows the force-velocity curves obtained for the fresh muscle and for the muscle at the end of the four fatiguing sequences. After the first sequence there was an increase in the velocity of the muscle contracting against the lightest load but, after this, the curve moved downwards and to the left as the muscle lost force and slowed. These changes could have been due to a loss of isometric force or to a change in the shape of the force-velocity curve.

To allow for the loss of isometric force the loads were expressed relative to the force of the isometric contraction (P/Po) in Fig 3b. The results for the last fatiguing sequence compared with the fresh muscle show the two curves to be diverging with a possible halving of the maximum velocity of shortening.

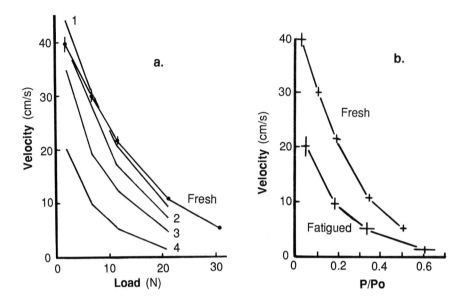

Figure 3. Force-velocity relationships for the adductor pollicis at rest and with the development of fatigue. **a.** Velocity of contraction as a function of load; results for fresh muscle and at the end of four fatiguing sequences (see text); values are mean ± SEM of 8 determinations for the fresh muscle and means of four determinations for the fatigue runs (one subject). **b.** Data for fresh muscle and after the 4th fatiguing sequence from Fig 3a replotted with load expressed as a fraction of isometric force (mean ± SEM for both).

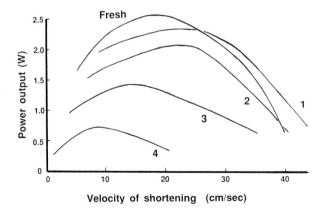

Figure 4. Changes in power output with developing fatigue. Power calculated from the results given in Fig 3a and plotted as a function of the velocity of shortening

How far can laboratory experiments explain the fatigue of athletes?

The power of each shortening contraction was calculated and Fig 4 shows the power output as a function of velocity for the fresh muscle and at the end of each of the four fatiguing sequences. This figure illustrates the early potentiation at the lowest loads, the progressive decrease in maximal power and the reduction in the velocity at which the maximum was obtained. The decrease in maximum power was associated with slowing of relaxation from the isometric tetanus. Values of maximum power taken from Fig 4 are plotted together with values of isometric force and relaxation (Fig 5). After the last sequence, the isometric force was reduced to about 60% of the fresh value while the power output was reduced to 30%. The divergence of isometric force and power coincided with the progressive slowing of the muscle relaxing from an isometric contraction.

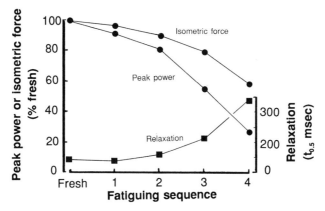

Figure 5. A comparison of the peak power, measured from Fig 4, and the force and half time of relaxation of the last isometric contraction of each fatiguing sequence.

Discussion

One of the main reasons for working on skeletal muscle fatigue is an interest in the factors which limit human performance, whether of an everyday nature or during competition. It has become apparent that there are major differences in the rates of fatigue during isometric contractions, mainly used in experimental work, and during dynamic exercise, which is of particular interest to the athlete.

Central fatigue
The limited experimental evidence available suggests that central fatigue during dynamic exercise is no more, and possibly less, of a problem than during sustained isometric contractions. The observation that central fatigue is less at higher speeds of contraction suggests that the inhibitory signals may arise from the forces generated in the muscle and tendons so that, at the higher velocities when force is less, there is less inhibitory input. This fact may explain the natural desire of most subjects, when pedalling a bicycle, to pedal faster as they fatigue. Although the dynamic contractions described here may be closer to "real life", the experimental arrangements are still very artificial and it remains to be seen whether afferent signals from working muscles affect the timing and coordination of the complex series of contractions which constitute whole body exercise. Most people who compete in athletic activity recognise that, as breathlessness and body temperature rise and pain in joints and legs becomes acute, timing and skill deteriorate and there is a reluctance to exercise further. Nonetheless to win a crucial point or avoid being overtaken on the line, the body can be forced into maximal activity. A tentative conclusion might be that central fatigue is important during everyday activities but, in times of crisis, or for the elite competitor, central fatigue *need not* be a limiting factor.

D.A. Jones

The energy requirements of dynamic exercise
In trying to explain the different rates of fatigue seen with various types of activity it is essential to know the energy costs of the exercise. Since the observations of Fenn (1923) it has been well known that more energy is liberated during shortening contractions than when a muscle is held at a constant length, but the majority of estimates of human muscle energy turnover have been based on isometric contractions or, occasionally, on submaximal working contractions. The results presented in Table 1 show that working contractions are twice as energetically demanding as sustained isometric contractions and this fact alone goes a long way towards explaining the very different patterns of fatigue illustrated in Fig 1. The present results were obtained with the muscle working close to its optimum loading for power output but a full understanding of the energetics of human muscle activity will require measurements to be made over the entire range of loads and velocities, including stretch, as well as estimates of the amounts of internal work done stretching tendons and ligaments. The most important aspect of dynamic muscle activity which has yet to be explored is the amount of recovery which can occur during and between working contractions. To maintain a given submaximal power output on a bicycle it is possible to pedal slowly and exert high forces or rapidly and exert low forces. The rapid movements would be expected to be more energetically demanding but, paradoxically, because of the lower forces, they may occlude the circulation to a lesser extent and allow the exercise to be continued for longer. This may be an alternative explanation for the natural desire of most people to increase pedal frequency as they tire.

Slowing of relaxation and loss of power during fatigue
The results shown in Fig 5 (together with the previous work of deHaan *et al*, 1989) suggest that slow relaxation and loss of power may be two symptoms of the same change occurring during fatigue.

The cause of slow relaxation is not known but there are two main possibilities. The first mechanism concerns calcium reaccumulation by the sarcoplasmic reticulum. Dawson *et al* (1980) found that changes in relaxation correlated with change in the affinity of ATP splitting and suggested that calcium pumping may be critically dependent on the free energy available from ATP. Allen *et al* (1989) have shown a prolonged calcium transient in muscle fibres fatigued to a point where they were relaxing slowly. Changes in calcium pumping, while possibly affecting relaxation from an isometric contraction, would not be expected to affect the cross bridge cycle or have any differential effect on force sustained during shortening contractions.

The second possible cause of slow relaxation is a reduced rate of cross-bridge detachment. This implies a change in the cross-bridge kinetics which should be reflected in the force-velocity curve of fatigued muscle much as has been found for animal and, now, human muscle. A reduction in ATP or an increase in ADP would both decrease shortening velocity by reducing the rate of detachment of the cross-bridge at the end of the power stroke but the concentrations at which these changes are seen (less than 1 mM ATP or about 4 mM ADP; Cooke & Bialek, 1979; Cooke & Pate, 1985) are most unlikely to occur in fatigued normal muscle. ATP is never likely to fall below about 4 mM or ADP rise above 0.5 mM. However, acidification of a muscle fibre, either as a result of fatigue or of manipulating the incubation medium, causes a reduction in the maximum velocity of unloaded shortening (Edman & Mattiazzi, 1981; Metzger & Moss, 1987; Chase & Kushmerick, 1988). The effect of the altered force-velocity relationship is to effectively change the muscle into a slower type of muscle with a reduced power output. Although the simple exponential form of relaxation suggests a single underlying biochemical process, evidence is accumulating that there are two processes which can cause slowing, one related to H^+ accumulation, the other being independent of pH change and probably dependent on a change in phosphorus metabolite levels (Cady *et al*, 1989b; Westerblad & Lannergren, 1991). It would be a pleasing coincidence to find that the pH dependent aspect was restricted to crossbridge function and that changes in phosphorus metabolites (within the physiological range) only regulate calcium uptake by the sarcoplasmic reticulum.

Summary
There are two features of dynamic contractions used during intense athletic exercise which set them apart from the sustained isometric contractions frequently studied in the laboratory. The first is the higher energy utilisation and the second is the greater sensitivity of shortening contractions to the metabolic changes which occur in exercising muscle. The combination of these two factors probably accounts for the rapid fatigue seen during maximal sprinting or cycling.

Acknowledgments: This work was supported by the Wellcome Trust and Medical Research Council. The muscle metabolite measurements are, as yet, unpublished results of work carried out with DB McIntyre, DL Turner & DJ Newham.

References

Allen DG, Lee JA & Westerblad H (1989) Intracellular calcium and tension during fatigue in isolated single muscle fibres from *Xenopus laevis*. *Journal of Physiology* **415**, 433-458.

Bigland-Ritchie B, Johansson R, Lippold OCJ & Woods JJ (1983) Contractile speed and EMG changes during fatigue of sustained maximal voluntary contractions. *Journal of Neurophysiology* **50**, 313-324.

Bigland-Ritchie B, Jones DA, Hosking GP & Edwards RHT (1978). Central and peripheral fatigue in sustained voluntary contractions of human quadriceps muscle. *Clinical Science* **54**, 609-614.

Cady EB, Jones DA, Lynn J & Newham DJ (1989a). Changes in force and intracellular metabolites during fatigue of human skeletal muscle. *Journal of Physiology* **418**, 311-325.

Cady EB, Elshove H, Jones DA & Moll A (1989b). The metabolic causes of slow relaxation in fatigued human skeletal muscle. *Journal of Physiology* **418**, 327-337.

Chase PB & Kushmerick MJ (1988) Effects of pH on contraction of rabbit fast and slow skeletal muscle fibres. *Biophysical Journal* **53**, 935-946.

Cheetham ME, Boobis LH, Brooks S & Williams C (1986) Human muscle metabolism during sprint running. *Journal of Applied Physiology* **61**, 54-60.

Cooke R & Bialek W (1979). Contraction of glycerinated muscle fibres as a function of MgATP concentration. *Biophysical Journal* **28**, 241-258.

Cooke, R & Pate E (1985). The effects of ADP and phosphate on the contraction of muscle fibres. *Biophysical Journal* **48**, 789-798.

Crow MT & Kushmerick MJ (1983). Correlated reduction in velocity of shortening and rate of energy utilization in mouse fast-twitch muscle during a continuous tetanus. *Journal of General Physiology* **82**, 703-720.

Dawson MJ, Gadian DG & Wilkie DR (1980) Mechanical relaxation rate and metabolism studied in fatiguing muscle by phosphorus nuclear magnetic resonance. *Journal of Physiology* **299**, 465-484.

deHaan A, Jones DA & Sargeant AJ (1989). Changes in velocity of shortening, power output and relaxation rate during fatigue of rat medial gastrocnemius muscle. *Pflügers Archiv* **413**, 422-428.

Edman KAP & Mattiazzi AR (1981) Effects of fatigue and altered pH on isometric force and velocity of shortening at zero load in frog muscle fibres. *Journal of Muscle Research and Cell Motility* **2**, 321-334.

Fenn WO (1923) A quantitative comparison between the energy liberated and the work performed by the isolated sartorius muscle of the frog. *Journal of Physiology* **58**, 175-203.

James C & Jones DA (1990) Changes in the isometric and dynamic force of fatigued human quadriceps muscle. *Journal of Physiology* **429**, 59P.

James C & Sacco P (1992) Central and peripheral fatigue during sustained dynamic exercise. *Journal of Physiology* (communication, in press).

Jones DA & Bigland-Ritchie B (1986). Electrical and contractile changes in muscle fatigue. In, *Biochemistry of Exercise VI*, ed. B. Saltin. International Series on Sports Sciences, Vol 16. Champaign, Ill., Human Kinetics Publishers. pp. 377-392.

Merton PA (1954) Voluntary strength and fatigue. *Journal of Physiology.* **123**, 553-564.

Metzger JM & Moss RL (1987) Greater hydrogen ion-induced depression of tension and velocity in skinned fibres of rat fast than slow muscles. *Journal of Physiology* **393**,727-742.

Newham DJ, McCarthy T & Turner J (1991) Voluntary activation of human quadriceps during and after isokinetic exercise. *Journal of Applied Physiology* **71**, 2122-2126.

Sargeant AJ, Hoinville E & Young A (1981) Maximum leg force and power output during short-term dynamic exercise. *Journal of Applied Physiology* **51**, 1175-1182.

Westerblad H & Lannergren J (1991) Slowing of relaxation during fatigue in single mouse muscle fibres. *Journal of Physiology* **434**, 323-336.

Fatigue and recovery of voluntary and electrically elicited dynamic force during cycling exercise in humans

A. Beelen, A.J. Sargeant, D.A. Jones* and C.J. de Ruiter

Department of Muscle and Exercise Physiology, Vrije Universiteit, Meibergdreef 15, 1105 AZ Amsterdam, The Netherlands, and Department of Physiology, University College London, Gower Street, London WC1E 6BT, U.K.*

Studies using electrical stimulation have shown that subjects are usually able to fully activate the quadriceps muscles in an isometric contraction including under conditions of fatigue (Bigland-Ritchie et al, 1978). It was not known whether this was also true for the main knee extensor muscles during maximal dynamic exercise involving a complex multi-joint movement as in cycling.

Methods

-*Force recording* : Force measurements were made during cycling on an isokinetic cycle ergometer in which the cranks were driven by an electric motor with a constant pedal frequency of 60 rev/min. Forces exerted on the pedals were monitored by strain gauges in the pedals.
-*Electrical stimulation* : During cycling the quadriceps muscles were stimulated transcutaneously through two 5 x 20 cm aluminium foil electrodes. The electrodes were applied proximally and distally on the anterior aspect of the thigh. Square wave pulses of $50\mu s$ duration were used at 200V. A train of 4 stimuli at 100Hz was delivered during 50ms. Stimulation of the resting quadriceps muscles in an isometric situation generated forces that were $36 \pm 9\%$ of the isometric MVC at the same knee angle.
-*Protocol*: : Fatigue was induced in 7 male subjects by a maximal sprint effort lasting 25s. Fatiguing exercise was performed on the iso-kinetic cycle ergometer at a pedal frequency of 60 rev/min. Before and after the sprint subjects allowed their legs to be passively taken round by the motor. During this passive movement the quadriceps were stimulated in order to generate peak stimulated force at 90° past top dead centre. The moment of stimulation was chosen such that peak stimulated force occurred at the same knee angle as the maximal voluntary force during maximal cycling exercise (Note this is a slightly different angle compared to the passive situation).

Forces generated by electrical stimulation of the passive muscle were determined before, and at intervals during the 20 minute recovery after the sprint. Measurements were made of the peak force and the maximum rate of force development as shown in figure 1.

Recovery of voluntary force was assessed in 4 subjects in a series of separate experiments in which, after recovery periods of different durations,.subjects performed a second maximal sprint effort

Results and Discussion

Peak stimulated force (PSF) immediately after the sprint was reduced to $69\pm3\%$ (Mean $\pm$SD). After 3 minutes recovery peak PSF had returned to pre-sprint values ($97\pm5\%$ of control). After about 5 minutes PSF reached 10% higher values compared to control. Thereafter stimulated force returned to control values (figure 2). The rate of force development was also reduced following the fatigue to $65\pm8\%$ of control and recovered with a similar time course as the peak stimulated force.

Voluntary force was reduced to $75 \pm 5\%$ of the control value at the end of the sprint but had fully recovered after 3 minutes ($98\pm3\%$ of control).

The association between the changes in stimulated force and voluntary force suggests that the fatigue in this type of dynamic exercise may be due to changes in the muscle itself and not to failure of central drive.

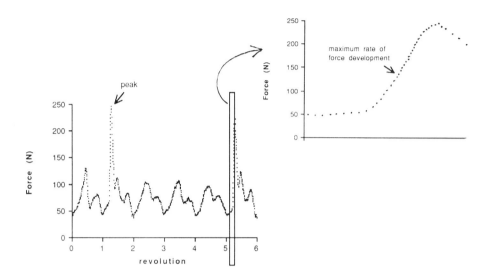

Figure 1. Example of force recording. Peak stimulated force and maximum rate of force development were calculated.

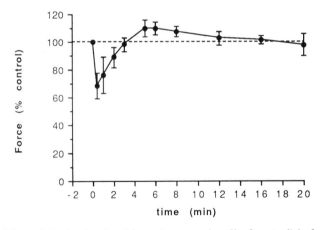

Figure 2.Peak stimulated force (expressed as % of control) before and at intervals during the recovery after the maximum sprint effort. Mean and SD of 7 subjects are given.

Reference

Bigland-Ritchie, B., Jones, D.A., Hosking, G.P., and Edwards, R.H.T. (1978) Central and peripheral fatigue in sustained voluntary contractions of human quadriceps muscle. *Clinical Science*. **54**, 609-614.

Shortening velocity, power output and relaxation rate during fatigue of skeletal muscle of young rats

A. de Haan, D.A. Jones* and A.J. Sargeant

Department of Muscle and Exercise Physiology, Faculty of Human Movement Sciences, Vrije Universiteit, Meibergdreef 15, 1105 AZ Amsterdam, The Netherlands.
* *Department of Physiology, University College London, United Kingdom*

Introduction

Muscle fatigue is usually assessed by the loss of isometric force, but in most daily activities skeletal muscles are used for movements and thus it is the maintenance of power which is important.

During sustained voluntary contractions muscle contractile properties change such that relaxation is slowed and contractions become more fused at lower frequencies. This acts to preserve force during isometric contractions (Bigland-Ritchie et al. 1972; Jones and Bigland-Ritchie 1986). It is not clear whether the slowing of relaxation also confers any advantageous effect on dynamic function. If the change in relaxation represents a prolongation of the active state due to slower reaccumulation of calcium into the sarcoplasmic reticulum, there is no obvious reason why this should affect the force-velocity characteristics of the whole muscle. If however the slowing is accompanied by a reduction in the rate of cross-bridge cycling, then a change in the force-velocity characteristics would be expected to result in lower force and therefore power output for a given velocity of shortening.

In the present investigation we have compared the loss of isometric force with that of maximal shortening velocity and power output during fatiguing contractions of rat medial gastrocnemius muscle. These changes occurring during fatigue have been related to changes in relaxation rate.

Methods

Young male Wistar rats (120 - 160g) were anaesthetized with pentobarbitone (60mg/kg; i.p.) and the medial head of the gastrocnemius was dissected free and distally attached to a force-transducer of an isovelocity measuring device (de Haan et al. 1989). Muscle temperature was maintained at 26°C by a water saturated airflow around the muscle. The most distal fibre bundle length was ~13mm and the length of the muscle belly ~25mm. The muscles were maximally stimulated (pulse heigh: 1mA; stimulation frequency: 60Hz) via the severed sciatic nerve.

The muscle was taken through a repeated cycle of alternative long (15s) and short (1s) contractions with 15min recovery after each long contraction and 5min after a short contraction. The muscle was first stretched to L_0 +2mm and then stimulated for either 1 or 15s. The muscle was released by 4mm at preset velocity, such that 0.3s before the end of stimulation the length was equal to L_0. To minimize the effect of elasticity we chose to measure the force attained after 3mm of release i.e. at L_0-1mm (F). F was expressed as a fraction of the isometric force immediately prior to release (F_0). The muscle was held at L_0-2mm while tension redeveloped until stimulation came to an end. The half time of relaxation was measured from the subsequent relaxation by taking the time needed for force to fall from one half to a quarter of the force reached at the end of stimulation.

A hyperbolic curve was fitted to the force and velocity data points using an iterative least squares method. The power-velocity curve was calculated from this fitted force-velocity curve.

Unloaded shortening velocity was determined using the "slack test" (Edman 1979). The sequence of events was similar to that used for the isovelocity releases, except that the amplitudes of the releases were 4, 5, 6, or 7mm at a nominal velocity of 500mm/s.

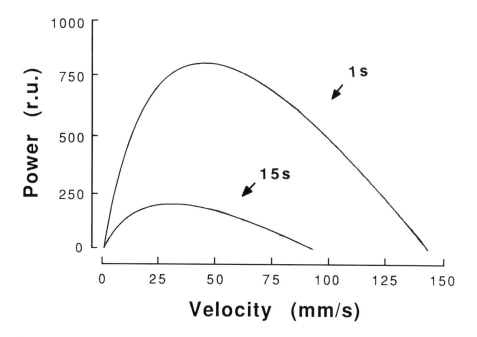

Figure 1. Power in relation to velocity for four muscles performing alternating long (15s) and short (1s) contractions. Power is given in relative units expressing force as a percentage of the peak isometric force attained in that contraction prior to shortening and velocity in mm/s for the complete muscle-tendon preparation.

Results and discussion

Following the 15s contraction the half time of relaxation was almost doubled and maximum shortening velocity reduced to ~64% compared to the 1s contractions. The data of the unloaded shortening velocity confirmed the reduction in maximal shortening velocity as estimated from extrapolation of the calculated force-velocity curve (Table 1; Fig.1).

Isometric force decreased to 48 ± 15% of the maximum during the fatiguing 15s contraction: However this reduction in isometric force greatly under-represented the loss of power. Due to the combination of reduced force and velocity of shortening, maximum power (at the velocity where power was greatest) decreased to ~24% following the 15s contraction. The reduction in power was even more pronounced at higher velocities (Fig.1).

The results are similar to those of Crow & Kushmerick (1983) and demonstrate that at a time when relaxation was slowed there was a change in the force-velocity relationship such that the normally fast medial gastrocnemius muscle assumed the characteristics of a slow muscle. The change in the force-velocity characteristics indicates a slower rate of cross-bridge turnover in fatigued muscles.

Thus the slowing of relaxation during fatigue can at least in part be attributed to a slowing of cross-bridge turnover. The results also demonstrate that isometric force may be a poor indicator of loss of performance in fatiguing exercise involving external work and power output.

Table 1. Summary of contractile properties of medial gastrocenemius muscles at the end of short and long contractions

	Short (1s) contractions	Long (15s) contractions
Unloaded shortening velocity. (mm/s)	143 (8)	88 (13)
Maximal shortenening velocity (mm/s)	145	93
Maximum power (relative units)	816	195
Velocity with maximum power (mm/s)	44.8	30.6
Half time of relaxation (ms)	11.9 (1.3)	20.6 (3.9)

Unloaded shortening velocity is given as the mean (SD) for 5 muscles.
The values for maximum shortening velocity, maximal power and velocity with maximum power are from the fitted curve in Fig. 1. Half time of relaxation is from the total number of contractions (24) from four muscles.

References

Bigland-Ritchie B, Johansson RS, Lippold ECJ and Woods JJ (1983). Contractile speed and EMG changes during fatigue of sustained maximal voluntary contractions. *Journal of Neurophysiology* **50**: 313-324.
Crow MT and Kushmerick MJ (1983). Correlated reduction in velocity of shortening and rate of energy utilization in mouse fast-twitch muscle during a continuous tetanus. *Journal of General Physiology* **82**: 703-720.
De Haan A, Jones DA and Sargeant AJ (1989). Changes in velocity of shortening, power output and relaxation rate during fatigue of rat medial gastrocnemius muscle. *Pflügers Archiv (European Journal of Physiology)* **413**: 422-428
Edman KAP (1979). The velocity of unloaded shortening and its relation to sarcomere length and isometric force in vertebrate muscle fibres. *Journal of Physiology* **291**: 143-159.
Edwards RHT, Hill DK and Jones DA (1975) Metabolic changes associated with the slowing of relaxation in fatigued mouse muscle. *Journal of Physiology* **251**: 287-301.
Jones DA and Bigland-Ritchie B (1986). Electrical and contractile changes in muscle fatigue. In Saltin B (Ed) *Biochemistry of Exercise VI*. Human Kinetics Publishers, Champaign, Ill., pp 337-392.

A. de Haan, D.A. Jones and A.J. Sargeant

Acid-base status during a graded field test related to marathon performance

J.A. Zoladz [1], A.J. Sargeant [2] and J. Emmerich [1]

[1] Department of Physiology and Biochemistry, Academy of Physical Education,
Al. Jana Pawla II 62a, 31-571 Cracow, Poland.

[2] Department of Muscle and Exercise Physiology, Faculty of Human Movement Sciences,
Vrije University, Meibergdreef 15, 1105 AZ Amsterdam, The Netherlands.

It is well documented that short term maximal exercise results in a decrease in muscle and blood pH. The resulting acidosis has been suggested to impair muscle function (Boyd et al. 1974, Sahlin 1986, Cooke et al. 1988).
However rather few data are available on the changes in acid-base status during high intensity exercise performed by top class, highly trained, athletes. In this paper data collected in a graded field test is presented for a group of runners with personal best marathon time in the range of 2:13:27 to 2:20:51.

Data is presented for a group of four top class male marathon runners who performed a graded field test within a few weeks of a marathon race. Additionally and for comparison, data for subject K.J. is included. This subject performed his last marathon 2 months prior to the test and significantly decreased his training programme during the intervening period. The graded field test was performed on an artificial running track. The test consisted of five separate bouts of running. Each bout lasted six minutes with an intervening 2 minutes rest period during which arterialized capillary blood samples were taken. Blood was analyzed for pH, pO_2, pCO_2 using the instrument Plastomed, Poland. The values of base excess (BE) and bicarbonate concentration (HCO_3^-) were calculated by this system. Lactate concentration was determined according to the method described by Barker and Summerson (1941) and modified by Strom (1949).
The exercise intensity during the test was regulated by the runners themselves by using the Sport Tester Polar Electro PE 3000 (Finland). The subjects were asked to perform the first bout of running at a constant heart rate (HR), which was 50 beats per minute below their individual maximal heart rate. Every subsequent bout, each of which lasted 6 minutes, was performed with an increment of 10 beats/min in the target HR. The mean velocity of each bout was then expressed for each individual in relation to their most recent marathon performance. Data is given as mean ± SD.

The average marathon velocity (vM) was 18.46 ± 0.32 km/h. On the basis of the formulas presented by Davies and Thompson (1979) we calculated that our runners at the speed corresponding to 100 % of vM had an oxygen uptake of 65 ± 1 ml/kg BW, which was approximately 84 % of VO_2max.
In the graded test there was a linear increase in heart rate with running velocity (p<0.02). No systematic changes in the blood acid-base status was observed until mean running velocity of the bout exceeded vM. In the bouts performed at velocities above vM there was a marked increase in lactate concentration and significant decrease in pH, HCO_3^- BE and pCO_2.
Thus in the last sub-vM bout in which mean velocity was 97 ± 0.8 % of marathon velocity blood pH was little changed compared with the rest value (mean value 7.36 ± 0.03 in both cases). In subsequent bouts at speeds above the mean marathon speed there was a marked and progressive fall in blood pH (fig.1).
The blood lactate concentration at a mean running velocity of 97.1 ± 0.8 % of vM was 2.33 ± 1.33 mmol/l which compares with a rest value of 1.50 ± 0.60 mmol/l was not significantly higher. However when running velocity exceeded the vM by only 3.6 ± 1.9 percent, the lactate concentration rose to 6.94 ± 2.48 mmo/l (p<0.05 vs.rest). The running velocity, associated with a fixed blood lactate concentration of 4 mmol/l in the group of four runners was estimated, by linear interpolation of the data, to be in the range between 97.8 to 102.1 % of the mean marathon velocity.

The results of the group of 4 top class marathon runners demonstrates that blood pH changes little in the bouts performed at running speed below 100% vM. However once vM was exceeded there was a marked change in acid base status. It is interesting to note the significant differences in the response of K.J. This runner had reduced his training in the period between the marathon and the graded test and blood pH during the test started to fall at some what lower relative velocities (%vM) compered with the group as a whole. (Figure 1.)

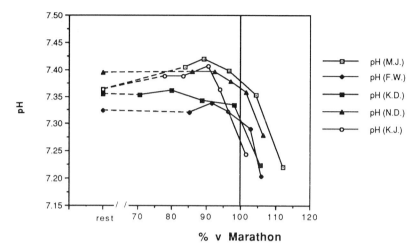

Figure 1. Blood pH levels in relation to running velocity during the graded test bouts, expressed as % of the mean marathon velocity.

Our data are in accordance with those published by Fohrenbach et.al. (1987), who found that at the end of a run of 45 min duration, at an intensity corresponding to the marathon velocity, no decrease in pH was observed when compared to the values at the 10th minute of exercise. In conclusion, it seems probable that these top class marathon runners run the marathon at highest velocity which can be sustained without a significant decrease in blood pH, although blood lactate concentration is already somewhat elevated.

Furthermore it seems that this form of graded field test may be a sensitive indicator of the training status for these runners as indicated by the quantitative changes seen in the responses of runner K.J. during a period of reduced training. As such, it may prove to be a valuable tool for optimizing training programmes.

The authors wish to thank Dr. J. Stoklosa and Mgr A. Zychowski for taking and analysing the blood samples and the runners for participating in this study.

References

Barker SB, Summerson WH (1941) The calorimetric determination of lactic acid in biological material. Journal of Biological Chemistry 138, 535-554.

Boyd AE, Giamber SR, Mager M, Lebovitz HZ (1974). Lactate inhibition of lipolysis in exercise man. Meatabolism 23, 531-542.

Cooke R, Franks K, Luciani GB, Pate E (1988) The inhibition of rabbit skeletal muscle contraction by hydrogen ions and phosphate. Journal of Physiology 359, 77-97.

Davies CTM, Thompson MW (1979). Aerobic performance of female marathon and male ultramarathon athletes. European Journal of Applied Physiology 41, 233-245.

Fohrenbach R, Mader A, Hollman W (1987) Determination of endurance capacity and prediction of exercise intensities for training and competition in marathon runners. International Journal of Sports Medicine 8, 11-18.

Sahlin K.(1986) Muscle fatigue and lactic acid accumulation. Acta Physiologica Scandinavica (suppl 556) 128, 83-91.

Strom G. (1949) The influence of anoxia on lactate utilization in man after prolonged muscular work. Acta Physiologica Scandinavica 17, 440-451.

Fatigability of mouse muscles during constant length, shortening, and lengthening contractions: interactions between fiber types and duty cycles

John A. Faulkner and Susan V. Brooks

Department of Physiology and Bioengineering Program, University of Michigan Medical School, Ann Arbor, MI 48109-0622, USA

Abstract

Our working hypothesis is that slow and fast fiber types have evolved for the performance of specific tasks: slow fibers for sustained force during isometric contractions and low velocity shortening and lengthening contractions and fast fibers for maximum power during a single contraction and for sustained power during high velocity shortening contractions. We tested this hypothesis by comparing the average force, sustained force and sustained power developed by slow soleus and fast extensor digitorum longus (EDL) muscles of mice during constant length, shortening, and lengthening contractions at increasing duty cycles. The duration of the contractions, amount of displacement, and velocity of shortening and lengthening were controlled and muscles were allowed to develop an appropriate force for a given duty cycle. For both muscles and each type of contraction, the average force developed during single contractions decreased as the duty cycle was increased. During constant length contractions, soleus muscles sustained a four-fold greater force than EDL muscles. Surprisingly, soleus muscles were not more proficient than EDL muscles at sustaining force or power during shortening contractions at the optimum velocity for the development of power by soleus muscles, whereas EDL muscles developed the greater sustained power when each muscle contracted at its own optimum velocity for power. During isovelocity lengthening contractions at 0.25 L_f/s, soleus muscles produced more than two-fold the sustained force, or power, of fast muscles. In general, the results are in good agreement with our working hypothesis.

Introduction

Traditionally, muscular fatigue is defined as "a failure to maintain the required or expected force" (Edwards in Porter & Whelan, 1981, pg.1). This definition reflects the reliance of previous measurements of fatigability on protocols involving isometric contractions (Porter & Whelan, 1981). Subsequently, the NHLB Institute Workshop (1990) defined muscle fatigue as "a condition in which there is a loss in the capacity of a muscle for developing force and/or velocity, resulting from muscle activity under load and which is reversible by rest". Although the latter definition incorporates the concept that the fatigued state *impairs* the ability of the muscle to develop both force and velocity (Metzger & Moss, 1987), the approach remains that of measuring a *failure to maintain* or a *loss in* force, velocity, or both. When exercising, even highly trained athletes tend to exercise at an intensity that can be maintained, rather than an intensity at which failure occurs.

For slow soleus and fast extensor digitorum longus (EDL) muscles of mice, the highest force that could be sustained during repeated constant length contractions and the highest power the could be developed during repeated isovelocity shortening contractions at optimum velocity for power were compared (Brooks & Faulkner, 1991). The stimulation frequency, duration, and, where appropriate, displacement and velocity of shortening of all contractions were chosen to facilitate the comparisons between slow and fast muscles under comparable conditions. Under these circumstances, the muscle developed a force appropriate for a given duty cycle. At each duty cycle, the average force equilibrated within the first minute and then could remain constant for up to 40 min. The coupling between energy input and energy output was too rapid to postulate a role for decreased calcium release or calcium sensitivity under these conditions. The level of force maintained was more likely based on the concentration of inorganic phosphate (Hibberd et al. 1985), hydrogen ion concentration (Metzger & Moss, 1987), or some interaction between the two. In keeping with the concept of a *graded exercise test* (Balke & Ware, 1959), the force or power were increased by increasing the train rate of the contractions, and consequently the duty cycle. Consistent with previous observations, during repeated isometric contractions, slow soleus muscles lost less average force than fast EDL muscles. Consequently, with increasing duty cycle, slow muscles sustained a greater force than fast muscles. Similarly, during repeated isovelocity shortening contractions at the optimum velocity for power for each muscle, gradual increments in duty cycle produced a more rapid loss in force by fast than slow muscles. In spite of the more rapid loss in force, the two-fold higher values for optimum velocity for the fast muscles resulted in fast muscles developing higher values than slow muscles for sustained power (Brooks & Faulkner, 1991).

During almost any total body physical activity, skeletal muscles will at various times remain at constant length, shorten, or be lengthened. The muscle performs a specific type of contraction dependent on the interaction between the force developed by the muscle and the load. If an equivalent or a fixed load is encountered, no change in length occurs; if the muscle force is greater than the load, the muscle shortens; and if the force is less than the load, the muscle is stretched. Since repeated shortening, isometric and lengthening contractions are performed habitually by skeletal muscles, our purpose was to compare the ability of slow and fast muscles to sustain force during each type of contraction during graded increases in the duty cycle. Our working hypothesis was that slow and fast fiber types have evolved for the performance of specific tasks: slow fibers for sustained force during isometric contractions and low velocity shortening and lengthening contractions and fast fibers for maximum power during a single contraction and for sustained power during high velocity shortening contractions. We recognize that although fibers may have adapted for the performance of specific types of contractions, each fiber type will under certain circumstances be recruited to perform each of the three types of contractions for varying periods of time. Such performances will on occasion result in fatigue, injury, or both (McCully & Faulkner, 1986). We tested the hypotheses that with increments in duty cycle compared with slow muscles, fast muscles will develop and sustain lower forces: a. during repeated constant length contractions, b. during isovelocity shortening contractions at the optimum velocity for power of slow fibers, and c. during isovelocity lengthening contractions with both slow and fast muscles at 0.25 L_f/s.

Experimental methods

Data were collected in situ on slow soleus and fast EDL muscles of SPF male CD-1 albino mice (Brooks & Faulkner, 1991). Mice (1 to 2 months of age) were anesthetized with sodium pentobarbitone (80 mg·kg^{-1}). The distal tendon of the soleus, or EDL, muscle was exposed. A 5-0 suture was tied around the tendon and the tendon was severed distally. The mouse was placed on a temperature controlled (35°C) plexiglass platform. The knee was pinned and the foot taped to the platform. The tendon was tied to the lever arm of a servomotor (Cambridge Tech, Inc., Model 300H or 305). A microcomputer interfaced with the servomotor controlled the direction, magnitude and velocity of each displacement. For both muscles, a frequency of 150 Hz appeared optimum for maintaining force and power during repeated contractions (Brooks & Faulkner, 1991). A frequency of 150 Hz produced an isometric force of 100% of maximum force (F_o) for soleus and ~85% of F_o for EDL muscles. Forces and displacements were displayed on a storage oscilloscope and sampled by a microcomputer during: a. constant length contractions which were preceded by a quick stretch, 10% of L_f and ~5 L_f/s for soleus and ~10 L_f/s for EDL muscles, designed to bring force rapidly to the level of F_o; b. shortening contractions which were through ~10% L_f at ~1.8 L_f/s, the optimum velocity for the development of power for soleus muscles; and c. lengthening contractions which were through ~10% of L_f at ~0.25 L_f/s to prevent contraction induced injury (McCully & Faulkner, 1986). The use of isovelocity shortening and lengthening contractions at the same velocities for slow and fast muscles allowed us to assess fatigue effects on force and velocity based solely in terms of the decrease in the force developed by the muscle. If fatigue caused a decrease in both force and velocity, the decrease in force during repeated isovelocity contractions reflects both aspects.

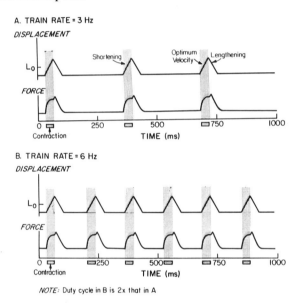

Fig. 1. Drawings of experimental records of repeated shortening contractions at two different train rates on identical time scales. Repeated contractions are at a train rate of 3 contractions/s (A) and at 6 contractions/s (B). Upper traces in both A and B show the displacements of the lever arm during isovelocity shortening and lengthening of the muscle. Displacement occurs around optimum length (L_o). Lower traces show the force developed. The stippled bars show the duration of stimulation which in this example occurs during shortening and is ~60 ms and ~30 ms for soleus and EDL muscles respectively (Modified from Faulkner et al. 1990 with permission).

Fatigability of mouse muscles

The concept of a test with graded increments of force or power was achieved through gradual increases in the train rate of repeated contractions (Brooks & Faulkner, 1991). During each cycle of contraction and rest, the fraction of time occupied by the contraction, termed the duty cycle, is equal to the product of the train rate in Hz and the contraction duration in seconds. For each experiment, the duration of each contraction was constant, therefore increments in the train rate and duty cycle were proportional. During each contraction, the average force was measured. To facilitate the comparisons among muscles of different masses, all measurements of force were normalized to specific force (N/cm^2) through division by the total cross-sectional area of the fibers. The mean values for specific F_o of 23.7 ± 0.9 N/cm^2 and 24.5 ± 0.7 N/cm^2 and muscle masses of 8.1 ± 0.4 mg and 8.9 ± 0.5 mg for soleus and EDL muscles respectively are in good agreement with previous data (Brooks & Faulkner, 1991). Sustained force was calculated as the average force developed during single contractions multiplied by the duty cycle. Protocols commenced at a train rate of 0.25 Hz and then the train rate was increased every five minutes with increments such that the value for sustained force increased with the increased duty cycle until a maximum sustainable value was reached. Drawings of records are shown in Figure 1 for repeated shortening contractions at two different train rates and therefore two different duty cycles. Similar records could be drawn for constant length and lengthening contractions.

Results

For both soleus and EDL muscles, the average forces during repeated constant length, shortening, and lengthening contractions decreased as a function of the increase in duty cycle. During constant length and lengthening contractions, the rate and magnitude of the decrease in average force relative to the duty cycle was greater for EDL than soleus muscles (Figure 2A, 2C). During contractions with both muscles shortening at the optimum velocity for the development of power by soleus muscles, soleus muscles never developed higher average forces than EDL muscles. Initially, the average force of EDL muscles was higher than that of soleus muscles. Subsequently, at high duty cycles, the average forces developed by EDL and soleus muscles were not different (Figure 2B). When the EDL muscle shortened at its optimum velocity, the average force developed was lower than the other two values (Figure 2B).

During each of the three types of contractions, the sustained force developed by soleus muscles increased substantially with increased duty cycle, whereas that of EDL muscles increased substantially only during shortening contractions (Figure 2A', 2B', 2C'). The sustained forces developed by EDL muscles increased only marginally with duty cycle during constant length contractions and not at all during lengthening contractions. During constant length, shortening, and lengthening contractions, the maximum values for the sustained forces of soleus muscles were 4.6 N/cm^2, 0.48 N/cm^2, and 2.9 N/cm^2, compared with 1.38 N/cm^2, 0.43 N/cm^2, and 1.31 N/cm^2 for the EDL muscle (Figure 2A', 2B', 2C').

The sustained powers developed by soleus and EDL muscles shortening at 1.8 L_f/s (the optimum velocity for power development by soleus muscles) were not different. In contrast, when each muscle shortened at its own optimum velocity for the development of power, the two-fold higher velocity of the EDL muscles resulted in higher sustained power outputs at almost every duty cycle (Figure 3). The soleus muscles did not sustain power well above a train rate of 3 Hz or a duty cycle of 0.18, whereas EDL muscles sustained power quite well up to a train rate of 10 Hz and a duty cycle of 0.3.

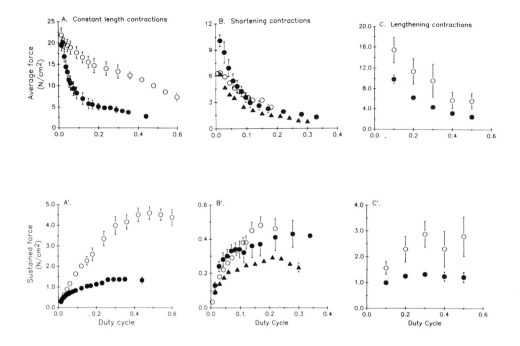

Fig. 2. The relationship of duty cycle with the average force (A, B, C) developed by slow (open symbols) and fast (filled symbols) muscles during the final (A) constant length contraction, (B) shortening contraction, and (C) lengthening contraction at each duty cycle. At each duty cycle, contractions are repeated for 5 min. The values for sustained force (A', B', C') were calculated from the product of average force and duty cycle. Each symbol represents the mean for 3 to 10 measurements. In panels B and B', circles indicate shortening at 1.8 L_f/s and triangles indicate 3.5 L_f/s. Error bars shown when 1 SEM is larger than the symbol (Modified from Brooks & Faulkner, 1991 with permission).

Discussion

Our observation that during repeated constant length contractions slow soleus muscles maintain higher average and sustained forces than fast EDL muscles is consistent with a number of previous reports that with repeated isometric contractions slow whole muscles (Segal et al. 1986) and motor units (Burke et al. 1973) are less fatigable than fast muscles or motor units. Our observation extends the range of duty cycles over which slow muscles demonstrate a superiority over fast muscles in developing force with less evidence of fatigue. The average specific force of fast muscles decreased rapidly as the duty cycle was increased above 0.025. At high (0.4 to 0.6) duty cycles, slow muscles had a four-fold greater average and sustained force than fast muscles. Presumably, the magnitude of the difference results from slow muscles having a greater oxidative capacity (Rigault & Blanchaer, 1970) and a lower energy requirement for the maintenance of a given force than fast muscles (Crow & Kushmerick, 1982). The data support the supremacy of slow over fast fibers for the performance of constant length

Fatigability of mouse muscles

contractions. The more rapid loss of average force by EDL muscles than by soleus muscles indicates that, compared with soleus muscles, EDL muscles experience a greater decrease in the number of attached cross-bridges, less force developed by each cross-bridge, or some combination of these two mechanisms. The present experiment does not permit the resolution of these options, nor the mechanism responsible for the change. In spite of these limitations, our data are consistent with the observations of Metzger & Moss (1990) that during isometric contractions at low pH, only fast fibers show a reduction in number of attached cross-bridges, whereas both slow and fast fibers show a decreased force per attached bridge.

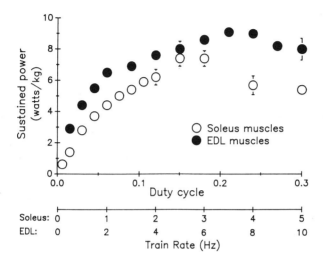

Fig. 3. The relationship between the sustained power and the duty cycle/train rate for slow soleus and fast EDL muscles. The power developed during each 5 min period at a given duty cycle was represented by the final cycle of activity and rest. The power sustained at each duty cycle was determined by multiplying the power developed during the final isovelocity shortening contraction by the duty cycle. The correspondence of the train rates and duty cycles assume a 60 ms and 30 ms contractions for soleus and EDL muscles respectively. Power (W) was normalized to wet muscle mass. Each symbol represents the mean for 6 to 10 measurements. Error bars shown when 1 SEM is larger than the symbol (Modified from Brooks & Faulkner, 1991 with permission).

In contrast to the differences in the average and sustained forces developed by slow and fast muscles during constant length contractions, slow muscles were not superior to fast muscles in developing and sustaining force when the shortening velocity for both was optimum for power development by the slow muscles. The lower than optimum velocity of shortening for the fast EDL muscles increased the average and sustained force developed, but reduced the power output compared to that developed at optimum velocity for a fast muscle (Brooks & Faulkner, 1991). In spite of the low velocity for the EDL muscles, during shortening contractions, the maximum sustained power outputs were not different for soleus and EDL muscles. The equivalence in the maximum sustained power output of slow and fast fibers at low velocities would enable muscles composed of slow and fast motor units to perform a variety of low velocity tasks with equal contributions of power from slow and fast motor units. In addition, fast oxidative motor units would be capable of performing high power tasks beyond the sustained power capabilities of slow motor units.

During stretches of activated single frog fibers, measurements of stiffness indicate that the number of attached cross-bridges is only about 10% to 20% greater than during an isometric contraction, indicating that the high forces observed during lengthening are due predominantly to increased strain of cross-bridges (Lombardi & Piazzesi, 1990). During lengthening contractions at low velocities, the two-fold greater average forces developed by soleus compared with EDL muscles likely reflects to some degree the two-fold higher elastic modulus of slow fibers (Metzger & Moss, 1990). The larger drop for fast muscles in the magnitude of average force with duty cycle indicates differences in the rate of fatigue between slow and fast muscles during lengthening contractions. Not only do the slow muscles sustain force better than fast muscles during lengthening contractions, but when the lengthening extends through greater displacements, the slow fibers are less likely to be injured than fast fibers (Jones et al. 1986).

The duty cycles that can be achieved with specific types of contractions reflect complex interactions between stimulation frequency, displacement, velocity, load, contraction duration and train rate. In addition, the duty cycle that can be sustained is dependent on the contractile history of the muscle. Only the lowest duty cycles could be sustained successfully from the resting state. Muscles that had been at rest had to progress through several increments of low duty cycles before the higher duty cycles could be sustained. Once muscles had achieved energy balance through several lower level duty cycles, subsequent duty cycles could be sustained for up to 40 min. In terms of the duty cycle achieved, the soleus muscles were superior to the EDL muscles during constant length contractions, whereas during shortening contractions, EDL muscles achieved higher duty cycles and train rates. Consequently, the duty cycles and train rates that can be tolerated place constraints on the tasks that muscles or motor units can perform. The tolerable levels have implications for stride, stroke, or pedalling frequency during various physical activities.

Acknowledgements This research was supported by a grant from the USPHS, National Institute on Aging AG-06157 and support to SVB on a Multidisciplinary Training Grant on Aging AG-00114.

References

Balke B & Ware RW (1959). An experimental study of "physical fitness" of air force personnel. *United States Armed Forces Medical Journal* 10, 675-688.

Brooks SV & Faulkner JA (1991). Forces and powers of slow and fast skeletal muscles in mice during repeated contractions. *Journal of Physiology* **436**, 701-710.

Burke RE, Levine DN, Zajak FE, Tsairis P & Engel WK (1973). Physiological types and histochemical profiles in motor units of the cat gastrocnemius. *Journal of Physiology* **234**, 723-748. et al., 1973

Crow MT & Kushmerick MJ (1982). Chemical energetics of slow- and fast-twitch muscles of the mouse. *Journal of General Physiology* **90**, 147-166.

Faulkner JA, Zerba E, & Brooks SV (1990). Muscle temperature of mammals: cooling impairs most functional properties. American Journal of Physiology 259 (Regulatory, Integrative, & Comparative Physiology 28): R259-R265.

Hibberd MG, Dantzig JA, Trentham DR & Goldman YE (1985). Phosphate release and force generation in skeletal muscle fibers. *Science* 228(4705), 1317-1319.

Fatigability of mouse muscles

Jones DA, Newham DJ, Round JM & Tolfree SE (1986). Experimental human muscle damage: morphological changes in relation to other indices of damage. *Journal of Physiology* **375**, 435-448.

Lombardi V & Piazzesi G (1990). The contractile response during steady lengthening of stimulated frog muscle fibres. *Journal of Physiology* **431**, 141-171.

McCully KK & Faulkner JA (1986). Characteristics of lengthening contractions associated with injury to skeletal muscle fibers. *Journal of Applied Physiology* **61**, 293-299.

Metzger JM & Moss RL (1987). Greater hydrogen ion-induced depression of tension and velocity in skinned single fibers of rat fast than slow muscles. *Journal of Physiology* **393**, 727-742.

Metzger JM & Moss RL (1990). Effects of tension and stiffness due to reduced pH in mammalian fast- and slow-twitch skinned skeletal muscle fibres. *Journal of Physiology* **428**, 737-750.

National Heart, Lung, and Blood Institute Workshop Summary (1990). Respiratory muscle fatigue. *American Review of Respiratory Disease* **142**, 474-480.

Porter R & Whelan J, Eds, (1981). *Human muscle fatigue: physiological mechanisms.* (Ciba Foundation Symposium 82) Pitman Medical. London.

Rigault MYA & Blanchaer MC (1970). Respiration and oxidative phosphorylation by mitochondria of red and white skeletal muscle. *Canadian Journal of Biochemistry* **48**, 27-32.

Segal SS, Faulkner JA & White TP (1986). Skeletal muscle fatigue *in vitro* is temperature dependent. *Journal of Applied Physiology* **61**, 660-665.

Force and EMG-changes during repeated fatigue tests in rat fast muscle

B.Zwaagstra, P.E.Voorhoeve and D.Kernell

Department of Neurophysiology, University of Amsterdam, Academisch Medisch Centrum, Meibergdreef 15, 1105 AZ Amsterdam, The Netherlands

Introduction

It is well known that, after common types of fatigue test, part of the recovery of force generation happens within seconds or minutes whereas other recovery processes are exceedingly slow (e.g. the 'low-frequency fatigue' of partly fused contractions; Edwards et al. 1977). This slow recovery, which may require several hours, makes it difficult to repeat tests in the same muscle or muscle unit for comparisons of the full fatiguing effects of different activity patterns. Hypothetically, fatigue processes of (moderately) rapid recovery characteristics ('fast-fatigue') might be studied separately in fatigue tests repeated at relatively brief intervals if:

(i) the initial fatigue test(s) could, as it were, be made to 'saturate' the fatigue process of slow recovery ('slow-fatigue') and

(ii) the recovery processes of slow- and fast-fatigue had widely different time constants.

Inspired by such ideas we explored whether, following initial 'priming' fatigue tests, moderately long test intervals in subsequent tests might evoke a constantly repeated pattern of fast-fatigue. Initial experiments indicated that a test interval of 20 min was too brief for a stationary result. The present report concerns repeated tests at 1 hr intervals.

Methods

The experiments were performed on the extensor digitorum longus muscle (EDL) of male adult rats (n=6; weights 320-380 g) anaesthetized with pentobarbitone. EDL was directly connected with a force transducer and kept at the optimum length for twitches. The muscle was activated via supramaximal electrical stimulation of muscle nerve. Electromyogram (EMG) was recorded via two bared thin wires thrust into the muscle belly. Nerve and muscle were covered with warm paraffine oil (36-38°C).

At intervals of 1 hr the following series of stimulations was repeated 6 times: (i) 10 single stimuli for evoking twitches; (ii) one burst of 200 Hz (duration 1 s) for evoking a maximum tetanic contraction; (iii) a fatigue test (cf. Burke et al. 1973) consisting of bursts of 40 Hz (duration 0.33 sec) repeated once a second for 4 minutes (totally 240 bursts). Peak forces were measured for contractions evoked by single or repetitive stimulation. All forces were expressed in relation (%) to that of the maximum tetanic contraction preceding the initial fatigue test ('test 1'). In the EMG, peak-to-peak amplitudes were measured for the evoked compound action potentials (M-waves).

Results and conclusions

The 1 hr test interval was sufficient for producing a full inter-test recovery of maximum tetanic force (Table 1). During test 1 there was a considerable initial force-potentiation (peak at around 20 s). This potentiation showed a very slow recovery; the peak force during potentiation was considerably smaller in tests 2-6 than in test 1 (Fig.1).

As seen during the *later* halves of consecutive fatigue tests, there was no progressive deterioration of force generation but rather, paradoxically, the contrary (Table 1, Fig.1). A qualitatively similar (and even more marked) tendency for a progressive increase was seen in the late EMG-reactions (Table 1).

Table 1. Contractile and EMG parameters per fatigue-test.
All force values expressed in per cent of the maximum tetanic force of test-1. EMG amplitudes (first M-wave per burst) given in per cent of M-wave amplitude for the first burst of test-1. Final force and EMG values refer to last burst of the respective fatigue test (i.e. value at 4 min after test start). Means±SD (n=6 tests).

Test no.	Tetanic force (%)	Twitch: Tetanus (%)	Final force (%)	Final EMG (%)
T-1	100	14.2±2.5	4.8±4.0	26.5±6.8
T-2	100±16	9.9±2.4	5.6±3.3	29.9±9.6
T-3	99±12	9.8±3.0	10.0±2.1	52.7±9.9
T-4	99±12	8.7±2.7	10.8±2.8	59.8±16.1
T-5	102±10	7.7±2.5	9.8±2.5	61.2±15.6
T-6	96±9	7.2±2.4	8.0±1.9	64.8±19.5

Following test 3, the force-reponses remained relatively similar during consecutive tests, particularly in later test-portions (Table 1, Fig.1). Simultaneously with these semi-stationary force responses during tests 3-6 there was, however, a significant progressive decrease in twitch amplitude (Table 1; paired t test for T-3 vs. T-6, $P < 0.01$).

The semi-stationary force-responses seen during the present kind of 'Burke-tests' repeated every 1 hr might provide a suitable background for testing the effects of different activation patterns on 'fast-fatigue'. It should be realized, however, that the apparently similar force-behaviour of fatigue tests 3-6 is likely to reflect a complex balance between several continuously changing parameters of importance for muscle force.

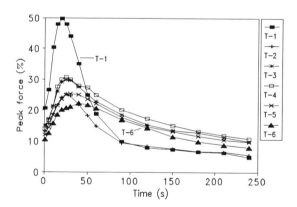

Figure 1. Time course of changes in peak burst force during consecutive fatigue tests (see T-1 to T-6 in symbol legend). All forces expressed in relation (%) to that for the maximum tetanic contraction preceding test T-1.

References

Burke RE, Levine DN, Tsairis P & Zajac FE (1973). Physiological types and histochemical profiles in motor units of the cat gastrocnemius. *Journal of Physiology* **234**, 723-748.

Edwards RHT, Hill DK, Jones DA & Merton PA (1977). Fatigue of long duration in human skeletal muscle after exercise. *Journal of Physiology* **272**, 769-778.

B. Zwaagstra, P.E. Voorhoeve and D. Kernell

Effect of an active pre-stretch on fatigue during repeated contractions

A. de Haan, M.A.N. Lodder and A.J. Sargeant

Department of Muscle and Exercise Physiology, Faculty of Human Movement Sciences, Vrije Universiteit, Meibergdreef 15, 1105 AZ Amsterdam, The Netherlands.

Introduction

Experiments performed using in situ mammalian muscles demonstrated that reduction of power consequent upon fatigue was more pronounced than the loss of isometric force (De Haan et al. 1988, 1989a). In those experiments the shortenings were preceded by an isometric force-generating phase. However, in activities such as running, many muscles of the lower extremities appear to be actively stretched before they are allowed to shorten. For such stretch-shortening cycles increased work output and efficiency were reported (Edman et al.1978; Heglund and Cavagna 1987). Higher muscle efficiencies during exercise might have consequences for the higher resistance to fatigue. Thus, in the present study we investigated whether changes in work output during a series of repeated contractions were affected by an active pre-stretch. Muscle contractions were compared in which shortening was preceded either by an active isometric phase or by an active stretch.

Methods

Medial gastrocnemius muscles of anaesthetized male Wistar rats (pentobarbitone 60mg/kg; i.p.) were stimulated (pulse height 1mA; stimulation frequency 60Hz) via the severed sciatic nerve (temperature 25°C). Force and displacement signals were A/D converted and fed into a microcomputer.

The muscles performed 10 repeated contractions ($1.s^{-1}$; duration 0.45s). Each contraction consisted of a pre-phase (duration 150ms) followed by a shortening phase lasting for 300ms (Fig. 1). During the shortening phase the muscle-tendon complex was allowed to shorten at a constant velocity ($20mm.s^{-1}$) from L_0 + 3mm to L_0 - 3mm, at which length stimulation was stopped and the muscle relaxed.

Six muscles were passively stretched and held at L_0 + 3mm. Stimulation was then begun and isometrically force developed for 150ms before the muscle was allowed to shorten (pre-isometric (PI) contractions). In the other six muscles activation was started while lengthening the muscle-tendon complex. The complex was actively stretched for 120ms (from L_0 + 0.6mm to L_0 + 3mm) with a velocity of $20mm.s^{-1}$, was subsequently remained isometric for 30ms, whereafter shortening was allowed (prestretch (PS) contractions; see Fig. 1).

Results and discussion

Force and work output
In the majority of previous studies on the effects of an active stretch, amphibian muscles have been stretched from an active isometric state (Katz 1939; Cavagna et al.1968; Edman et al.1978). However, as stated by Asmussen and Bonde-Petersen (1974) the onset of activation in vivo seems to take place in the last phase of the stretch. Moreover, Heglund and Cavagna (1987) reported that efficiency of rat EDL muscle was highest when the stretch commenced just before the onset of activation The present protocol showed that when stimulation was started during lengthening of the muscle-tendon complex a more than twofold enhancement in force could be achieved (see Fig.1). At L_0 + 3mm in the PI experiments the isometric peak force was ~60% of the isometric force obtained at L_0 (mean ± SD: 11.0 ± 0.8N; n=12); in contrast the peak force in the PS contraction was 150% of the isometric force at L_0 (Fig. 1).

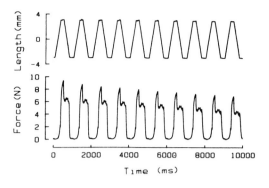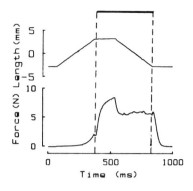

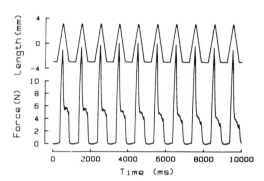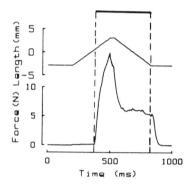

Figure 1. Examples of force and length traces obtained during series of pre-isometric contractions (top diagrams) and prestretch contractions (bottom diagrams).

<u>Left:</u> series of 10 successive contractions.

<u>Right:</u> enlarged diagrams of the first contraction of the series. The upper black bars indicate the time of stimulation.

Length is given relative to muscle optimum length (L_o).

Taken over the whole 10 contractions, the total work output during the shortening phase of the PS group was ~40% higher compared to the PI group (354 ± 36 vs. 254 ± 49mJ). The *extra* total work output of the PS group was predominantly (~70%) produced during the first 100ms of the shortening, while only 7% of the extra work was produced in the last 100ms of the shortening. This indicates that recoil of series-elastic elements had a large contribution in this *extra* work output.

Fatigue

The absolute difference in work output between the first and tenth contraction was not different for the PI and PS groups (9.53 ± 2.73 and 9.55 ± 1.93 mJ), respectively). This could imply that the contribution of the active contractile component (i.e. cross-bridge cycling) to work output in the shortening phase, and thus the time course of fatigue, was not affected by pre-stretch. All the extra work output performed after an active stretch would then originate from sources other than cross-bridge cycling and these sources would be hardly or not at all sensitive to fatigue. The findings that energy utilization was not affected by prestretch (De Haan et al.1989b, 1991) is in keeping with this hypothesis.

The changes in forces immediately prior to shortening were quite different for the PI and PS contractions (Fig.2). Whereas the force during the series of PI contractions decreased by 2-3% per contraction, the force after an active stretch (in the PS group) increased by ~8% in the first

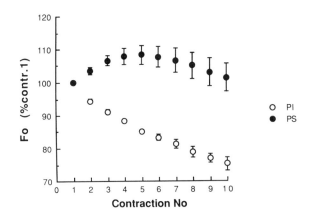

Figure 2. Relative changes in the force immediately prior to shortening for the series of 10 pre-isometric (PI) and prestretch (PS) contractions.
Mean (SD; n=6) for force (Fo) is given relative to the force of the first contraction of the series (=100%).

4 contractions before declining by ~1% per contraction. This is consistent with the observation of Curtin and Edman (1989) who noted a relatively smaller fatigue effect on force during active stretching of single fibres.

As a consequence of the similar absolute reductions in work output with the number of PI and PS contractions, the relative reduction (which is how fatigue is often expressed in human physiology) was less after a prestretch (26% vs 32%). Thus prestretch gives the impression of apparently protecting against fatigue.

References

Asmussen E and Bonde-Petersen F (1974). Storage of elastic energy in skeletal muscles in man. *Acta Physiologica Scandinavica* **91**: 385-392.

Cavagna GA, Dusman B and Margaria R (1968). Positive work done by a previously stretched muscle. *Journal of Applied Physiology* **24**: 21-32.

Curtin NA and Edman KAP (1989). Effects of fatigue and reduced intracellular pH on segment dynamics in isometric relaxation of frog muscle fibres. *Journal of Physiology* **413**: 159-174.

De Haan A, Van Doorn JE and Sargeant AJ (1988). Age-related changes in power output during repetitive contractions of rat medial gastrocnemius muscle.*Plfügers Archiv (European Journal of Physiology)* **412**: 665-667.

De Haan A, Jones DA and Sargeant AJ (1989a) Changes in velocity of shortening, power output and relaxation rate during fatigue of rat medial gastrocnemius muscle. *Pflügers Archiv (European Journal of Physiology)* **413**: 422-428.

De Haan A, Van Ingen Schenau GJ, Ettema GJ, Huijing PA and Lodder MAN (1989b). Effifiency of rat medial gastrocnemius muscle in contractions with and without an active prestretch. *Journal of Experimental Biology* **141**: 327-341.

De Haan A, Lodder MAN and Sargeant AJ (1991). Influence of an active pre-stretch on fatigue of skeletal muscle. *European Journal of Applied Physiology* **62**: 268-273.

Edman KAP, Elzinga G and Noble MIM (1978). Enhancement of mechanical performance by stretch during tetanic contractions of vertebrate skeletal muscle fibres. *Journal of Physiology* **281**: 139-155.

Heglund NC and Cavagna GA (1987). Mechanical work, oxygen consumption and efficiency in isolated frog and rat muscle. *American Journal of Physiology* **253**: C22-C29.

Katz B (1939). The relation between force and speed in muscular contraction. *Journal of Physiology* **96**: 45-64.

The design of the muscular system

Lawrence C. Rome

Department of Biology. University of Pennsylvania. Philadelphia, PA 19104 USA

Abstract Animals produce a wide range of movements, both fast ones and slow ones. Many parameters in the muscular system (maximum velocity of shortening [V_{max}], gearing of fibers, kinetics of activation and relaxation, myofilament lengths) show considerable variation. Our goal has been to determine the rules (design constraints) which govern what values these parameters have in a given animal. By a combination of whole animal measurements during locomotion (sarcomere length [SL] changes, muscle shortening velocity [V], and fiber recruitment) and isolated muscle mechanics measurements (V_{max}, SL-tension relationship), we have found evidence for two constraints in the design of the muscular system. Parameters appear to be set so that 1) active fibers operate over optimal myofilament overlap (where maximum tension is generated) and 2) active fibers shorten at V/V_{max}'s of 0.17-0.38 (where maximum power and optimal efficiency are obtained). A given animal produces a wide range of movements while its active fibers obey these constraints, by recruiting different fiber types that have different V_{max}'s and different gearing (Δ body movement/Δ SL). Because different fiber types also have different metabolic capabilities, these mechanical constraints have important implications for neuromuscular fatigue.

One of the most fascinating areas of physiology is the study of how parameters of a given system are fine-tuned to provide optimal performance under a variety of conditions. The components that make up the muscular system are fairly well understood and some show tremendous variation. It seems reasonable that evolution has set the values of various parameters to enable animals to locomote over a wide range of speeds efficiently.

Although we know what the important components are and how they vary, we do not know how the system is designed. An understanding of how the muscular system is designed requires us to understand how the various components are integrated into the system, or more specifically, given the variation that occurs in each component, by what rules does evolution choose the values for each parameter.

Over the past seven years, my laboratory has performed both isolated muscle and whole animal experiments in a effort to elucidate (1) whether there are identifiable rules by which values for various components of the system are set to enable animals to perform the wide range of activities that a given animal performs and (2) whether or not these rules hold for the great variety of locomotory behaviors in which vertebrates engage.

From cell physiology, we may anticipate that there are some rules (Fig.1) that are followed when an animal muscular system is designed. During steady activation, the force muscle generates depends on the amount of overlap between myosin and actin filaments, or more precisely, the number of myosin crossbridges which can interact with actin sites (Gordon et al.1966). It would seem sensible for animals to vary the gear ratio of their muscle fibers and their myofilament lengths, so that no matter what movements the animal makes, the muscle would operate at optimal myofilament overlap (i.e. where the muscle generates near maximal force). As such, gear ratio and myofilament lengths can be viewed as the design parameters (those components that can be varied during evolution). Myofilament overlap can be viewed as a design constraint or design goal (i.e., what has to remain constant or the rule by which the variation in parameters is adjusted). As both design parameters are anatomical features of the muscle, one at the organ level and the other at the molecular level, this can be viewed as a structural design consideration.

There is also a dynamic design consideration which takes into account that muscle shortens

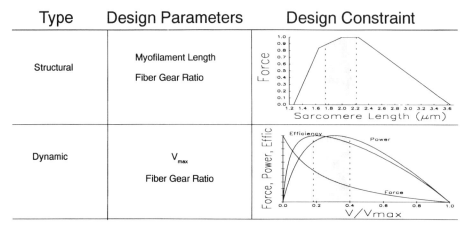

Type	Design Parameters	Design Constraint
Structural	Myofilament Length Fiber Gear Ratio	
Dynamic	V_{max} Fiber Gear Ratio	

Figure 1. Steady state design constraints. Our empirical studies suggest that myofilament overlap and V/V_{max} are important design constraints, that is, the rules by which the values of design parameters are set.

during locomotion. The force muscle generates is a function of V/V_{max}. More importantly, the mechanical power that a muscle generates and the efficiency with which it generates the mechanical power are functions of V/V_{max} as well. Again, we might anticipate that the muscular system would be designed so that no matter what movement the animal makes, the active fibers operate over a range of V/V_{max} values (0.15 - 0.40), where the fibers generate maximal power at maximum efficiency. Thus, the design parameters V_{max} and fiber gear ratio are varied in such a way that they operate under the design constraint of V/V_{max}.

Different types of animals face very different problems during locomotion and hence, their muscles must perform different activities. Because the potential design constraints listed above formally refer only to shortening contractions (as opposed to isometric or lengthening contractions), our research to test these design constraints has focused on animals which primarily use shortening contractions (fish and frogs).

I. Design Constraint #1 - Myofilament overlap

The simplest design constraint is myofilament overlap (the SL-tension relationship). Because of the sliding filament structure of muscle, muscle generates maximum force over a fairly narrow range of SLs (Gordon et al.1966). Researchers have assumed that the muscle is used only over those SLs, but there has been relatively little evidence to justify this assumption.

Our recent experiments on carp provide the most extensive study of these issues. To swim, a fish must bend its backbone. By a combination of high speed motion picture and anatomical approaches, we have found that at low swimming speeds, the red muscle (Fig. 2), which powers this movement, undergoes cyclical SL excursions between 1.89 to 2.25 μm centered around a sarcomere length of 2.07μm (Rome et al.1990a). Further, we determined from electron microscopy that thick and thin filament lengths of the red (1.52μm and 0.96μm) and white (1.56μm and 0.99μm) muscle in carp are similar to that in frogs (Sosnicki et al.1991). Using the frog SL-tension relationship, the red muscle was shown to be operating over a range of SLs where no less than 96% maximal tension is generated (Rome and Sosnicki, 1991).

We then examined the most extreme movement carp make, the escape response. This involves a far greater curvature of the backbone than steady swimming. If the red muscle were powering this movement, it would have to shorten to a SL of 1.4 μm where low forces and irreversible damage can occur (Fig 2c; Rome and Sosnicki, 1991). Rather it is the white muscle which performs the movement, because the white muscle has a different orientation than the red. The red muscle fibers run parallel to the long axis of the fish just beneath the skin (Fig. 2a). The white muscle fibers on the other hand, run in a helical orientation with respect to the long axis of the fish. We have empirically shown that the helical pattern

The design of the muscular system

endows the white muscle with the a 4-fold higher gear ratio (Δ backbone curvature/ΔSL).

Thus, for a given backbone curvature, the white muscle undergoes only about 1/4 the SL excursion of the red. To power this most extreme movement of fish, in the worst case (posterior), the white muscle must shorten to a SL of 1.75μm (Fig. 2c). At this SL the muscle generates about 85% maximal force. Most of the volume of the white muscle (middle and anterior sections), however, does not shorten as much and thus generates even more force (95% for anterior and 92% for the middle). When the white muscle is used in less extreme movements (i.e., during fast swimming), the curvature of the backbone is not nearly as severe, and thus the white muscle generates nearly maximal force (Rome and Sosnicki, 1991).

As we have shown above, the myofilament overlap is never far from its optimal level even in the most extreme movements. It appears, therefore, that animals are designed in such a way that no matter what the movement, the muscles used generate nearly optimal forces. As such, myofilament overlap can be considered a design constraint (i.e., an aspect of the system that is kept constant). Given the movements that animals need to make, two design parameters (fiber orientation and myofilament lengths) are adjusted during evolution such that the active fibers always operate at near maximal myofilament overlap and force generation (Fig. 1).

To test this design constraint further, we examined frog jumping. It seemed that in an all-out movement like a frog jump, a good strategy might be to circumvent (to some extent) this constraint and for the frog to passively stretch the sarcomeres to long lengths in its crouching position. Hence, instead of being restricted to small SL excursions (as in fish), the sarcomeres could shorten up the descending limb, through the plateau, onto the shallow ascending limb, providing a longer SL change (stroke) and produce more work.

Lutz and Rome (1991) have recently shown on two hip extensor muscles (gracilis and semimembranosus) that frogs in fact do this. During a jump, both muscles shorten from a resting sarcomere length of ~2.6μm down to ~2.0μm. Over these SL's the muscle would generate no less than 75% maximum force. However, at the point in the jump when the frog is generating maximum power (~2.38 μm), the force would be no less than 91%. These results further support the theory that myofilament overlap is a design constraint in muscular systems, although it is a slight variation on the theme evidently adapted for jumping.

II. Design Constraint #2-V/V$_{max}$

V_{max} can vary greatly. Differences in V_{max} have been found in a given muscle at different temperatures, in different muscle fiber types within the same muscle, and in muscles from different animals. To a first approximation, fibers with different V_{max}'s generate the same maximum isometric force per cross-section and have the same maximum efficiency, whereas the maximum power generated and rate of ATP splitting in the fiber with a high V_{max} is considerably greater than in the fiber with a low V_{max} (Fig. 3).

From Hill's work (Hill, 1938), we know, however, that a muscle fiber's mechanical properties (force generation and power production) and energetic properties (ATP utilization and efficiency) are not simply a function of the fiber's V_{max}. They also depend on V/V_{max}.

Figure 3 shows the force, power output, and efficiency of fibers with 2 different V_{max} values. For a given V, the force and mechanical power per cross sectional area can be considerably higher in the fiber with a high V_{max} (at V_1, they are similar, whereas at V_2, they are quite different; Fig. 3a,b). It would thus seem advantageous to only have muscle fibers with high V_{max}'s. There is, however, an energetic price paid for a high V_{max}. The rate of ATP utilization in the fiber with a high V_{max} is considerably greater than in a fiber with the low V_{max} at all velocities of shortening. Thus, there appears to be an adaptive balance between the mechanics and energetics of contractions. The fibers with low V_{max} are more efficient at low V (e.g. V_1). At higher velocities (e.g. V_2), however, the fibers with high V_{max} are more efficient (Fig 3c). Thus, to produce both slow movements and fast movements efficiently, the animal should use the fibers whose V_{max} is matched to the V at which it needs to shorten.

If V/V_{max} is in fact a design constraint we would anticipate that a given muscle fiber type would be used over a range of V/V_{max} of about 0.15 to 0.40 where efficiency and power output are maximal. Thus the two design parameters, V_{max} and gear ratio, should be set so that during all body movements, the V falls within this range of V/V_{max} (as in Fig. 1).

To determine V/V_{max} one must determine (1) which muscle fibers are active during a given activity, (2) the V at which the fibers shorten (i.e, slope of the SL-time graph), and (3) the V_{max} of the different fiber types. It is the first of these measurements which led us to work on

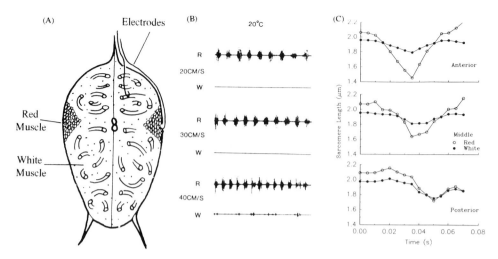

Figure 2. Cross-sectional view of carp (a). The red muscle forms a thin sheet just under the skin (its thickness is exaggerated for illustrative purposes). The red fibers run parallel to the body axis (i.e., out of the page). The white fibers run in a helical fashion with respect to the backbone. Consequently, they need shorten by only ~1/4 as much as the red ones to produce a given curvature change of the body. Placement of electromyography (EMG) electrodes are shown. EMGs from red (R) and white (W) muscle of carp at 20°C (b). The SL excursions of the white muscle in the anterior, middle and posterior positions during the startle response (c). Note that the red fibers do not actually shorten to the SL shown because they cannot shorten fast enough. Adapted from Rome et al. (1984,1988) and Rome and Sosnicki, (1991).

fish. Because of the anatomical separation of their different muscle fiber types (Fig 2a), it is possible to monitor activity of different fiber types by EMG. For instance, we know from EMGs at slow speeds that only the red fibers are active, and at fast speeds the white muscle fibers are recruited as well (Fig. 2b).

To test the importance of V/V_{max} as a design constraint, we have examined this parameter in four situations. Each situation was chosen to change either the numerator, V, or the denominator, V_{max}, in order to see if there was a concomitant change in the other parameter to maintain a constant V/V_{max}.

A. Different Fiber Types in Carp

The first question we asked is why animals have different fiber types (i.e., different V_{max}'s within the same animal). Are the faster fibers used for faster movement (higher V's) so that they operate at the same V/V_{max}? As illustrated in Fig. 3, the V_{max} of carp red muscle was 4.65 muscle lengths/s (ML/s) and the V_{max} of carp white muscle 2.5 times higher, 12.8 ML/s (Rome et al.1988). During steady swimming the red muscle is used over ranges of velocities of about 0.7 to 1.5 ML/s (shaded portion of Fig. 3d). This corresponds to a V/V_{max} of 0.17-0.36, where maximum power is generated. At higher swimming speeds (higher V's) the fish recruited their white muscle because the mechanical power output of the red muscle declines.

It is clear from Fig. 3d, that red muscle cannot possibly power the escape response. To power the escape response, the red muscle would have to shorten at 20 ML/s, which it clearly cannot do, as this is 4 times its V_{max}. But even if the white muscle were placed in the same orientation occupied by the red (i.e., same gear ratio), it couldn't either, because its V_{max} is only about 13 ML/s. However, because of its 4-fold higher gear ratio, the white muscle need shorten at only 5 ML/s to power the escape response (Fig. 3), which corresponds to a V/V_{max} of about 0.38, which is where white muscle generates maximum power.

Thus the red and white muscle form a two gear system which powers very different movements. The red muscle powers slow movements, while the white muscle powers very fast movements, both while working at the appropriate V/V_{max}. In terms of backbone curvature, the white muscle can produce 10-fold faster movements (2.5-fold higher V_{max} x 4

The design of the muscular system

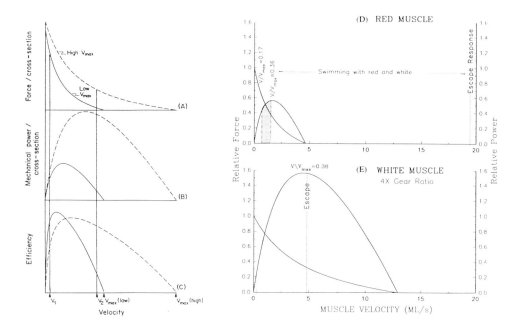

Figure 3. Relative force (a), power (b), and efficiency (c) as a function of relative shortening velocity for a muscle with a high V_{max} (dashed curves) and a muscle with a low V_{max} (solid curves). V_1 and V_2 are arbitrarily chosen examples of low and high shortening velocities. Design constraint #2--V/V_{max} (d,e) During slow movements and fast ones the <u>active</u> fibers always shorten at a V/V_{max} of 0.17-0.38 where maximum power and efficiency are generated. During steady swimming (red muscle), the fibers are used at a V/V_{max} of 0.17-0.36 (d). The red fibers cannot power the escape response because they would have to shorten at 20 ML/s. The escape response is powered by the white muscle which need shorten at only 5 ML/s (V/V_{max} =0.38) because of its 4X higher gear ratio (e). The white muscle would not be well suited to power slow swimming movements, because it would have to shorten at too low a V/V_{max} (0.01-0.03; adapted from Rome 1990,1992).

-fold higher gear ratio).

There also appears to be a minimum V/V_{max} at which fibers are used. For instance, if the white muscle does so well producing fast movements, why doesn't the fish have only one fiber type and let the white muscle power the slow swimming movements as well? The white muscle could certainly power slow swimming, but it is not used because its high V_{max} and 4-fold higher gear ratio would make its V/V_{max} at slow swimming speeds too low (i.e., 0.01-0.03, where the muscle is nearly isometric and efficiency is nearly 0; see shaded portion of Fig. 3e). At slightly faster swimming speeds, when the white muscle starts to be recruited to augment the power of the red, if the fish were to continue swimming steadily, the white muscle would still be shortening with too low a V/V_{max} to generate power efficiently. Under these circumstances, however, the fish employs "burst and coast swimming" in which it makes rapid tail beats (i.e., short duty cycle) with the white muscle to obtain a high V and to keep an optimal V/V_{max}. At very slow swim speeds, (i.e., to the left of the shaded portion in Fig. 3d), carp also use the "burst and coast" pattern, but this time with the red muscle. This allows the fish's red muscle to make the normal SL excursion in less time (shorter duty cycle) resulting in normal V/V_{max} and efficiencies. Thus carp adopt a "burst and coast" pattern of swimming when the muscle fiber type being used would have too small a V/V_{max} to generate power with a high efficiency if the fish were swimming steadily (Rome et al. 1990a).

Thus given the constraints at both high V/V_{max} and at low V/V_{max}, to achieve a full repertoire of movement, animals must use different fiber types with different V_{max}'s and different gear ratios. It should be further recognized that these "mechanical" constraints indirectly set the level of activity at which neuromuscular fatigue occurs. The white fibers have a low mitochondrial density and a low capillarity. Thus they have little ability to consume oxygen to replenish high energy phosphate stores. When swimming speed increases such that anaerobic fibers must be recruited to generate the requisite mechanical power (i.e., V/V_{max} of the red muscle becomes too high), the ATP used will be supplied anaerobically. This leads to white muscle lactate accumulation and glycogen depletion, and ultimately to fatigue. Therefore, swimming speeds at which anaerobic fibers are recruited are not sustainable (Rome et al. 1984). These mechanical constraints also explain the onset of neuromuscular fatigue at lower speeds at cold temperatures (see next section).

B. Different Muscle Temperatures in Carp

Raising the temperature of a muscle increases its V_{max}. If V/V_{max} is an important design constraint, then the animal should use its muscle over a higher range of V's at the higher temperatures. Indeed, the V_{max} of carp red muscle is 1.6-fold greater at 20°C than at 10°C (Rome and Sosnicki, 1990). Although at a given swimming speed, the V at which the muscle shortens is independent of temperature, carp at 20°C could swim to 45 cm/s with the red muscle exclusively, while at 10°C they could only swim to 30 cm/s (Rome et al.1990a). Hence, the corresponding V at the respective maximum speed was 1.6-fold higher at 20°C than at 10°C (2.04 vs 1.28 ML/s respectively), resulting in the same V/V_{max} (0.36) at both temperatures. In addition, the 10°C fish could swim steadily at lower speeds than at 20°C, corresponding to a 1.6-fold lower V (resulting in the same V/V_{max} at the lowest speed). Thus at both 10 and 20°C, carp use their red muscle over the same range of V/V_{max} (0.17-0.36).

C. Fast swimming species (scup) vs slow species (carp)

At a given temperature, the marine scup can swim twice as fast with its red muscle as the fresh water carp (80 cm/s vs 45 cm/s at 20°C; Rome et al.1992a). We anticipated that the scup's maximum V (i.e., while swimming at 80 cm/s) would be twice as high as the carp's maximum V (i.e. while swimming at 45 cm/s). If maintaining V/V_{max} is important, then the V_{max} of scup should be twice as high as the carp's as well.

Remarkably, because scup employ a less undulatory style of swimming than carp (i.e. smaller backbone curvature and smaller SL excursion), at their respective maximum swimming speeds with red muscle, the V's at which the muscles shorten are equal (about 2.04 ML/s; Rome et al.1992a). We now expected carp and scup red muscle should have the same V_{max}, which is exactly what we found (Rome et al.1992b). Hence, both the fast fish and the slow fish use their red muscle over the same V/V_{max} (0.17-0.37) even though it corresponds to much higher swimming speed in scup.

D. Scaling of V_{max} with Body Mass (M_b) in Mammals

Although the muscles in mammals perform a variety of activities in addition to shortening (active lengthening and remaining isometric; Goslow et al.1981), V/V_{max} appears to be important in this muscle as well. Stride frequency at physiologically equivalent speeds scales with $M_b^{-0.16}$ (where M_b is body mass; Heglund and Taylor, 1988). As SL excursion may be independent of M_b, V should scale with $M_b^{-0.16}$ as well. Hence, the V in large animals should be much lower than in small ones, and thus to maintain a constant V/V_{max}, the large animals should have a much lower V_{max}. The V_{max} of large animals had never been previously measured largely for technical reasons. We developed single fiber histochemistry techniques and combined them with myosin light and heavy chain electrophoretic techniques to enable us to differentiate the 3 major fiber types (Sosnicki et al.1989). We then used single skinned fiber mechanics techniques, and measured V_{max} of three fiber types within the horse soleus muscle (Rome et al.1990b). The mean V_{max} varied over 10-fold between fiber types, which presumably provides the horse with the flexibility to power a wide range of motor activities.

By comparing V_{max} measured on the horse to that previously measured on the rat and on the rabbit, we examined scaling of V_{max} over a 1200-fold size range (Rome et al.1990b). The V_{max} of slow oxidative fibers (SO, Type I) scaled with $M_b^{-0.18}$ which is close to the $M_b^{-0.16}$ for stride frequency and V, suggesting that the SO fibers of large and small animals operate over the same V/V_{max} and at similar efficiencies. Fast glycolytic fibers (FG, Type IIb), on the other hand, scaled with $M_b^{-0.07}$, and thus FG fibers have a higher V_{max} in large animals than needed for maintaining a constant V/V_{max}. FG fibers, however, are likely used infrequently, only when the horse is jumping or running at maximum speed. In this case the horse might be

The design of the muscular system

willing to sacrifice efficiency for increased mechanical power provided by a higher V_{max}.

E. Summary of steady state design constraints

Thus, in four different cases which might lead to changes in V/V_{max}, evolution has taken the appropriate measures to maintain a constant V/V_{max}. In the three fish experiments, V/V_{max} is between 0.17 and 0.38, where power and efficiency are maximal (Fig. 1), showing that V/V_{max} is an important design constraint. The way animals produce a wide range of movements is by using fibers with different V_{max}'s and with different gear ratios. In the case of mammals, it appears that V_{max} scales appropriately to maintain a constant V/V_{max}, but it is not known precisely what this value is.

In conclusion, it appears that animals use their muscles over a narrow range of myofilament overlaps and over a narrow range of V/V_{max} where muscle generates maximum force and maximum power with optimal efficiency (Fig. 1). Therefore during evolution, three design parameters (gear ratio, V_{max} and myofilament lengths), appear to have been adjusted so as to obey these design constraints no matter what movement is made. Hence, these design constraints appear to be two of the rules by which muscular systems have been put together.

III. Non-steady state constraints

Although V/V_{max} and myofilament overlap appear to be important design constraints, they may not represent a complete description of muscle behavior during locomotion. The problem is that these constraints are based on the force-velocity and SL-tension curves, which are measures of steady state mechanics of <u>maximally</u> activated crossbridges. In this type of experiment, the muscle is stimulated at a fixed length (isometric) and is allowed to shorten only after generating maximum tension (indicating complete activation). The muscle is then given several minutes to relax (complete relaxation) prior to being relengthened and stimulated again. Although these steady state measurements are useful for studying the mechanics of contraction, this is not how the muscle is used during locomotion and thus may ignore other important constraints on muscle design. Unlike the steady state experiments, during cyclical locomotion muscle fibers alternately activate and relax and shorten and lengthen with no time delay in between (Josephson, 1985).

Intuitively it seems beneficial that fibers be fully "activated" during shortening and fully "relaxed" prior to relengthening. If the muscle were able to instantaneously activate and instantaneously relax then the mechanical behavior during shortening could be well described by steady state properties of muscle. Although during very low oscillation frequencies, muscle activation and relaxation requires a small fraction of the cycle and hence can be viewed as instantaneous, during oscillation frequencies that animals <u>actually use</u> during locomotion, the muscle may run into some important limitations.

Because the muscle cannot instantaneously relax (i.e., all the bridges detach so that subsequent lengthening of the muscle does not produce force), the muscle may have to operate in such a way that <u>deactivation proceeds during shortening</u> (Marsh, 1990). This could be achieved by cutting off the stimulus before the end of shortening and by an intrinsic property of the muscle called "shortening deactivation". If so, the crossbridges will not be maximally activated and force and power production will be below that described by the steady state force-velocity curve. In addition, incomplete relaxation would result in negative work. These competing effects are quantified by the net power during a complete cycle, which is equal to:

(work done by muscle shortening **- work done on muscle** lengthening**) per cycle x cycle freq.**

From these considerations we anticipate that net power output during swimming may involve a complex interplay between different muscle properties. Thus, the effect of activation-relaxation kinetics on the mechanical behavior of muscle <u>depends greatly on the conditions</u>.

There is relatively little known about whether during locomotion the kinetics of activation and relaxation impinge on the mechanical performance of the muscle. The basic problem is that this can only be discerned by imposing the exact length changes and stimulation pattern the muscle undergoes <u>in vivo</u> on isolated muscle, and measuring force production. However, this has <u>never been done before</u>.

We have recently taken a first step toward this goal by imposing on isolated muscle <u>in vivo</u> length changes and oscillation frequencies and the <u>in vivo</u> stimulus duty cycle (measured from

EMGs). At 20°C, muscle bundles run under these in vivo conditions produced nearly maximal power, suggesting that the muscle works optimally during locomotion (Rome and Swank, 1992). This also suggests that the kinetics of activation and relaxation as well as crossbridge kinetics have been adjusted to produce maximum mechanical power at the oscillation frequencies and length changes that scup need to use during swimming. Further work using this approach will be useful in elucidating the design constraints of activation and relaxation.

Acknowledgments: This work was support by NIH grant AR38404

References

Gordon, A. M., Huxley, A. F. & Julian, F. J. (1966). The variation in isometric tension with sarcomere length in vertebrate muscle fibers. *Journal of Physiology* **184**, 170-192.

Goslow, G. E., Seeherman, H. J., Taylor, C. R., McCutchin, M. N. & Heglund, N. C. (1981). Electrical activity and relative length changes of dog limb muscles as a function of speed and gait. *Journal of Experimental Biology* **94**, 15-42.

Heglund, N. C. & Taylor, C. R. (1988). Speed, stride frequency and energy cost per stride: how do they change with body size and gait? *Journal of Experimental Biology* **138**, 301-318.

Hill, A. V. (1938). The heat of shortening and the dynamic constants of muscle. *Proceedings of the Royal Society of London B* **126**, 136-195.

Josephson, R. K. (1985). Mechanical power output from striated muscle during cyclic contraction. *Journal of Experimental Biology* **114**, 493-512.

Lutz, G. & Rome, L. C. (1991). Design of frog muscle for jumping. *American Zoologist* **31**(5), 123A.

Marsh, R. L. (1990). Deactivation rate and shortening velocity as determinants of contractile frequency. *American Journal of Physiology* **259**, R223-R230.

Rome, L. C., Loughna, P. T. & Goldspink, G. (1984). Muscle fiber recruitment as a function of swim speed and muscle temperature in carp. *American Journal of Physiology* **247**, R272-R279.

Rome, L. C., Funke, R. P., Alexander, R. M., Lutz, G., Aldridge, H. D., Scott, F. & Freadman, M. (1988). Why animals have different muscle fibre types. *Nature* **355**, 824-827.

Rome, L. C. (1990). The influence of temperature on muscle recruitment and function in vivo. *American Journal of Physiology* **259**, R210-R222.

Rome, L. C., Funke, R. P. & Alexander, R. M. (1990a). The influence of temperature on muscle velocity and sustained performance in swimming carp. *Journal of Experimental Biology* **154**, 163-178.

Rome, L. C., Sosnicki, A. A. & Goble, D. O. (1990b). Maximum velocity of shortening of three fibre types from the horse soleus: Implications for scaling with body size. *Journal of Physiology* **431**, 173-185.

Rome, L. C., Choi, I., Lutz, G. & Sosnicki, A. A. (1992a). The influence of temperature on muscle function in fast swimming scup. I. Shortening velocity and muscle recruitment during swimming. *Journal of Experimental Biology* **163**, 259-279.

Rome, L. C., Sosnicki, A. A. & Choi, I. (1992b). The influence of temperature on muscle function in the fast swimming scup. II. The mechanics of red muscle. *Journal of Experimental Biology* **163**, 281-295.

Rome, L. C. & Sosnicki, A. A. (1990). The influence of temperature on mechanics of red muscle in carp. *Journal of Physiology* **427**, 151-169.

Rome, L. C. & Sosnicki, A. A. (1991). Myofilament overlap in swimming carp. II. Sarcomere length changes during swimming. *American Journal of Physiology* **260**, C289-C296.

Rome, L. C. & Swank, D. (1992). The influence of temperature on power output of scup red muscle during cyclical length changes. *Journal of Experimental Biology* **Submitted**.

Sosnicki, A. A., Lutz, G. J., Rome, L. C. & Goble, D. O. (1989). Histochemical and molecular identification of fiber types in single, chemically skinned equine muscle cells. *Journal of Histochemistry and Cytochemistry* **37**, 1731-1738.

Sosnicki, A. A., Loesser, K. & Rome, L. C. (1991). Myofilament overlap in swimming carp. I. Myofilament lengths of red and white muscle. *American Journal of Physiology* **260**, C283-C288.

Section V

Neuronal Mechanisms and Processes

Neuromuscular fatigue and the differentiation of motoneurone and muscle unit properties

D. Kernell

Department of Neurophysiology, University of Amsterdam, Academisch Medisch Centrum, Meibergdreef 15, 1105 AZ Amsterdam, The Netherlands.

Abstract It is well known that muscles consist of motor units with widely varying contractile properties. In the present survey an analysis is given of various ways in which the properties of the motoneurones are matched to those of their muscle units such as to help to minimize the risk for neuromuscular fatigue. This seems essentially to be done in two ways: (i) by matching the recruitment threshold of motoneurones to the fatigue-resistance of their muscle units, thus ensuring an appropriate choice of units for various types of motor task (*posture vs. movement match*); (ii) by matching the repetitive discharge properties of the motoneurones to those of their muscle units in ways that will serve to keep muscle units active, as much as possible, at low relative force levels (includes a *rate gradation match* between the minimum maintained firing rate of motoneurones and the contractile speed of their muscle units). Experiments with long-term stimulation of muscles suggest that part of the normally obtained matching between motoneurone and muscle unit properties may be caused and maintained by long-term effects of neuromuscular activity on muscle fibre properties (including endurance). In connection with the experiments on chronic stimulation it was noted that changes in fatigue sensitivity of muscles did not consistently occur in parallel with changes in the electromyographic behaviour of these muscles during fatigue tests.

Introduction

In the present context, neuromuscular fatigue will simply be defined as a decline of force taking place during a steady pattern of activation of some kind. Whether neuromusclar fatigue develops in a particular usage situation will depend on the combination of at least four major factors:

- (i) the properties and organization of the *muscle fibres* themselves, determining their fatigue-resistance (endurance) in various usage-contexts;
- (ii) the *kind of contraction* produced by the muscle fibres (isometric, concentric, excentric), depending on the force-balance between the target muscle, other muscles and external influences;
- (iii) the manner in which the fibres are activated by their *motoneurones* during the particular usage concerned;
- (iv) the extent to which the metabolic needs of the muscle fibres are adequately taken care of by relevant external supporting mechanisms (e.g. *(micro-)circulation, respiration, etc.*).

Below I will give a rather general survey centred on data concerning point (iii), i.e. I will primarily review in which ways the properties and the functional organization of the motoneurones are differentiated to make them handle their various brands of muscle units such that fatigue problems might be minimized. There are at least two obvious manners in which the motoneuronal management of muscle units may serve to decrease the risk for fatigue:

- (iii-a) by using an appropriate *muscle unit selection*, i.e. chosing the right unit for the right task (*recruitment optimalization*);
- (iii-b) by using an appropriate *level of muscle unit drive*, i.e. essentially by keeping the activation level (impulse rate) of each unit as low as feasible for a given usage situation (*frequency optimalization*).

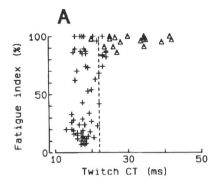
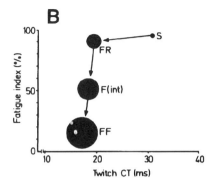

Figure 1. Graphs illustrating the co-variation between different contractile properties among muscle units of cat's peroneus longus muscle. Fatigue index (%) plotted versus twitch time-to-peak (ms) for 80 individual units (**A**) and for average values of the same units after categorization into types S, FR, F(int) and FF (**B**). In **B**, the diameter of each symbol is proportional to the maximum tetanic force of the respective unit category (mean force for FF units: 27.9 g). Reproduced with permission from Kernell et al. (1983) (**A**) and Kernell (1986) (**B**).

I will start by discussing the questions relating to muscle unit selection and that implies that I will first have to deal with a muscular problem, namely the normal degree of variability in contractile muscle unit properties (i.e. the functional range over which motoneurones might select different muscle units). With respect to muscle units as well as motoneurones, my overview will be illustrated with examples from our own experimental work, which has largely been performed on hindlimb muscles of cats and rats.

Normal pattern of co-variation among muscle unit contractile properties

It is well known that, within the average limb muscle of commonly used experimental animals, there is a characteristic pattern of co-variation between the maximum force, speed and endurance of the muscle units. This is illustrated by Fig.1, which shows the typical 'inverted L-shape' for the relation between measures of endurance and isometric speed (cf., however, less marked co-variation and smaller endurance-range among human thenar motor units; Thomas et al. 1991). In **A** individual values are shown; these data illustrate that there is essentially a *continuous* variation among the muscle units in their physiological properties. In **B** the various units have been categorized, for descriptive purposes, into the four classes S, FR, F(int), FF as defined by Burke and coworkers (see Burke et al. 1973; Burke 1981). At one extreme of the distribution we have units that are weak, slow and highly resistant to fatigue. At the other extreme, the units are fast and strong and of low endurance.

The endurance data of Fig.1 emanate from measurements with the *Burke-type fatigue test :* 0.33 sec stimulation-bursts of 40 Hz were repeated once a sec for 2-4 min, and a fatigue index was calculated which essentially corresponded to the fraction of initial burst-force still being produced after 2 min test activation (y-axes of Fig.1). It should be noted that this test was originally designed for classification purposes, and it might then be considered as an advantage that the test tends to produce a bimodal distribution of fatigue indices (bimodality sometimes much more marked than in Fig.1, cf. Burke et al., 1973). Part of this bimodality is apparently the result of a 'saturation' of endurance-values at the upper end of the distribution; FR or S units with similarly high fatigue indices according to a Burke-test may be demonstrated to differ considerably in endurance according to other tests (Botterman & Cope 1988; Cope et al. 1991). Furthermore, in a more long-lasting series of contractions than that of the typical Burke-test, the maintenance of force generation generally tends to be markedly better for S units than for FR units (cf. Burke et al. 1973; Botterman & Cope 1988).

Optimalization of motoneuronal recruitment: 'Property-ranked recruitment' and the 'posture vs. movement match'

In most motor acts, the muscle units tend to become recruited in the general order indicated by the arrows in Fig.1B, i.e. in the sequence S ➔ FR ➔ F(int) ➔ FF. On average, this will be a recruitment in an order of increasing unit force and that does, of course, correspond to one aspect of the 'size principle' of Henneman (review: Henneman & Mendell 1981). This principle was originally formulated on basis of experiments in which the measurements concerned an aspect of *motoneuronal* size, namely the relative diameter of the motor axon, which is often monitored in terms of axonal conduction velocity. As measured over the whole range of motoneuronal and muscle unit properties both components tend to co-vary in relative 'size', i.e. there is typically (at least in the cat) a positive correlation between axonal conduction velocity and muscle unit maximum force (particularly evident for S+FR units; e.g. Emonet-Dénand et al. 1988). Also *within* single classes of units (at least for the S units), recruitment tends to occur in order of increasing axon size (Bawa et al. 1984).

Intracellular measurements from our own as well as from other laboratories have suggested that intrinsic differences in motoneuronal electrical excitability are important for the commonly appearing recruitment hierarchy (e.g. Kernell 1966; Kernell & Monster 1981; Fleshman et al. 1981; Gustafsson & Pinter 1985): weaker currents are needed for the activation of small-axoned slow-twitch motoneurones than for the fast-twitch ones with larger axons. The relatively high excitability of the slow-twitch small-axoned cells is mainly caused by the relatively high specific resistance of their membrane (for references and further discussion, see Kernell 1992). Thus, there is seemingly no obligatory linkage between the motoneuronal (or axon) size and the motoneuronal (recruitment) excitability, and this kind of co-variation is also not universally present. One of the best-documented 'aberrations' is of particular relevance for neuromuscular endurance: at least for motoneurones of some muscles of the cat's hindlimb, the size vs. excitability correlation is absent when comparing fast-twitch cells of fatigue-sensitive (FF) and fatigue-resistant (FR) units. These axon and cell body sizes vary over the same range for FR and FF cells in spite of the fact that the FR motoneurones have a markedly higher average degree of electrical excitability (i.e. lower electrical current needed for activation; Fleshman et al. 1981; Kernell & Monster 1981), presumably mainly caused by their higher input (and specific membrane) resistance (Fleshman et al. 1981; for further discussion and references, see Kernell 1992).

It should be stressed that one of the most important and general messages contained in the concept of Henneman's 'size principle' is that recruitment typically takes place in a functionally adequate relation to the various contractile properties of the muscle units (e.g. Henneman & Mendell 1981; see further comments below); this remains valid also for cases in which aspects of motoneuronal size show little co-variation with other functional properties. There is a need for a more general term than 'size principle' when referring to motoneuronal behaviour in which the recruitment hierarchy is ordered in relation to contractile unit properties (but not necessarily in relation to axon size); one possibility would be the term *'property-ranked recruitment'* (Kernell 1992).

When analyzing the functional relevance of relationships between motoneuronal recruitment and muscle unit properties it is useful to consider them as representing two major types of motoneurone vs. muscle unit match (Fig.2):

- (a) The match between recruitment hierarchy (ascending-force-order of recruitment) and muscle unit maximum force represents a *'recruitment-gradation match '*. This match primarily serves to optimize the smoothness of force gradation by letting strong units be used mainly in muscle contractions of high total muscle force; thereby the *relative* force-magnitude of each recruitment step will be minimized (Henneman & Mendell 1981).

- (b) The match of recruitment hierarchy vs. fatigue-resistance and speed represents an endurance-related association, a *'posture vs. movement match'*. Posture is typically maintained by contractions of weak to moderate force and potentially very long duration. The units that primarily will become engaged in the execution of such contractions are the easily recruited S units. The high endurance of these units makes them, of course, eminently suited for postural tasks. Furthermore, the slow contractile speed of the S units would be of particular value in postural near-isometric contractions because the maintenance of force takes place at less metabolic expense in slow than in faster muscle (e.g. Crow & Kushmerick 1982). On the other hand, very strong contractions that mobilize much of the total resources of a muscle might mainly be needed for the transient acceleration phase of rapid movements and, in this situation, the fast contractile speed (and great power capacity) of the late-recruited FF units would clearly be of value. In strong

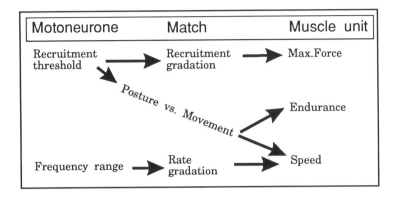

Figure 2. Scheme illustrating commonly occurring types of matching between motoneuronal behaviour and muscle unit properties.

contractions, capillaries will become compressed by surrounding activated muscle fibres and the local blood supply will become minimal or absent; hence, the poor oxidative capacity of fibres characteristic for FF units (cf. Burke 1981) might not matter much in their typical usage situations. On the other hand, it should be remembered that these 'fatigue-sensitive' fibres have a potentially relatively *high* endurance under ischaemic conditions because the anoxic metabolism of glycogen is more effective in fibres of type IIB (typically FF units) than in those of type I (typically S) (for refs., see Burke 1981).

The two recruitment-related matches of Fig.2 are to some degree potentially independent of each other, i.e. there is no obligatory linkage between the maximum force of a muscle unit and its speed or fatigue resistance. The extent to which all these three contractile properties tend to co-vary would be expected to be related to, for instance, the degree to which a particular muscle is actually used for postural support and/or rapid movement, thus motivating the appropriate kind of 'posture vs. movement match' between recruitment behaviour and endurance/speed-related unit properties. Maintained postural contractions are likely to be largely produced by S units. Hence, for instance, in the hindlimb it is appropriate that the percentage of S units indeed tends to be higher for the post-tibial anti-gravity muscles of the ankle than for their counterparts on the pre-tibial side (see literature-data compiled in Table 3 of Kernell et al. 1983).

Optimalization of motoneuronal discharge frequency

In muscles consisting of mammalian twitch fibres, it is of major importance for the gradability of force as well as for the realization of an endurance-promoting 'frequency optimization' that the muscle is not commanded by a single neurone but by a *multi-unit motoneurone pool*. The twitch elicited by a single action potential is often quite large in comparison to the maximum tetanic force (twitch vs. tetanus ratio commonly 0.15-0.30) and, if a whole muscle were managed by a single command-neurone, a smooth and steady level of contraction would only be obtained by activation rates high enough to cause near-fusion. However, the use of such nearly-fused contractions would be quite ineffective from various other points of view: endurance would low, circulation would be ineffective, and there would be little or no possibility for grading the force. In mammalian twitch muscle, the only way to combine a smoothness of force production with a reasonable degree of endurance and gradability of tension is to subdivide the muscle into different units that can be active *asynchronously* to each other. Thus, one might say that the evolutionary 'invention' of the twitch muscle fibre would in itself have produced sufficient motivation for a subsequent invention of the motoneurone pool as a commanding device (if not already invented for other reasons).

Slow and faster muscle units differ in the range of stimulation rates needed for the effective modulation of force (steep portion of tension-frequency curve), and the slow and faster motoneurones show corresponding differences in their intrinsically possible range of discharge rates. This represents a third kind of match between motoneuronal and muscle unit features, a *'rate-gradation match'* (Fig.2). Of particular relevance in this context is the minimum rate of maintained firing, i.e. the rate at which a neurone will tend to start firing when just barely recruited. This rate depends to an important extent on the time course of the post-spike afterhyperpolarization (AHP), which is of a duration about equal to that of the twitch (Kernell 1983; Bakels & Kernell, in preparation); besides the AHP, other factors may contribute as well to the setting of the minimum rate (cf. Carp et al. 1991). The rate-gradation match is typically such that, on recruitment, muscle units tend to start firing at discharge rates slow enough to produce almost completely unfused contractions (for references, see Kernell 1992). In maintained submaximal contractions, fatigue commonly develops less rapidly at low total forces than at higher output levels (Bigland-Ritchie & Woods 1984; Botterman & Cope 1988; Cope et al. 1991; cf. also Garland et al. 1988). Thus, for such reasons, the rate-gradation match is presumably important for the maintenance of an optimum degree of neuromuscular endurance during motor functions.

Differences in the minimum rate of maintained firing (as caused by differences in AHP duration) are of interest also in relation to yet another aspect of motoneuronal rhythmic behaviour: the frequency-adaptation. During the long-lasting intracellular activation of a motoneurone with a steady injected current, discharge rate declines continuously during at least the initial 1/2 - 1 minute of firing (Kernell & Monster 1982a). The precise mechanisms producing this *'late adaptation'* are still uncertain; AHP-related factors are not necessarily involved. For a given motoneurone, the late adaptation is more marked the higher the rate of firing at the onset of the discharge. When comparing different motoneurones that were activated by the same weak amount of suprathreshold current, the starting rate was (as expected) found to be lower in motoneurones of slow-twitch units and, correspondingly, these slow motoneurones also showed less late adaptation (Kernell & Monster 1982b). Thus, the slow-twitch motoneurones seemed particularly well suited for the production of steady postural contractions. In discharges at higher force levels and impulse rates, the late adaptation might in itself help to produce an endurance-promoting optimalization of discharge frequency. During the course of maintained contractions there is often a progressive slowing of contractile speed (Bigland-Ritchie & Woods 1984), and in relatively strong contractions the highest degree of average force output is actually produced by a steadily *declining* activation rate (Jones et al. 1979), such as is also seen to occur during the initial minute of a maximum voluntary contraction (Bigland-Ritchie & Woods 1984). Experimental evidence indicates that, in voluntary contractions, much of this rate decline is produced by reflexes (Woods et al. 1987; see also present symposium: Bigland-Ritchie, Gandevia, Stuart & Callister). The intrinsic motoneuronal properties associated with the late adaptation would, however, be likely to add to the rate drop as well, thereby in certain situations helping to minimize neuromuscular fatigue. In other cases, the late adaptation might conceivably instead *contribute* to central aspects of neuromuscular fatigue (see discussion in Kernell & Monster 1982b).

So far I have only talked about recruitment- and rate-gradation separately. Normally, these two strategies of force modulation are used in parallel, although their coupling may differ quantitatively between different muscles. The relative contribution from either one of the two mechanisms over a certain force range (cf. Milner-Brown et al. 1973) has to do with the balance between the ease of recruitment gradation ('recruitment gain', cf. Kernell & Hultborn 1990) and the ease of rate gradation (steepness of slope for relation between discharge rate and intensity of activating synaptic (or injected) current; cf. Kernell 1992). Over the range of weak muscle forces used for postural control it would be advantageous to have the motoneurones discharging at frequencies relatively close to their minimum rates because: (i) the first-recruited units tend to be slow-contracting, having a comparatively limited frequency-range for the rate-modulation of force; (ii) low relative rates and unit tensions would generally be expected to promote endurance. A preponderance of relatively slow rates might be attained by having the thresholds of consecutively recruited neurones close to each other, thus allowing but little rate gradation to take place in parallel with the recruitment of additional cells. If such a close spacing of recruitment thresholds were primarily dependent of intrinsic motoneuronal properties (i.e. as opposed to synaptic distribution, cf. Kernell & Hultborn 1990), one would expect to find more densely clustered intracellular current-thresholds for the 'postural' S-motoneurones than for the more movement-associated FR or FF cells. Our data for intracellularly investigated rat and cat motoneurones have shown that this is also actually the case (Bakels & Kernell, in preparation; cf. data of Kernell & Monster 1981; Fleshman et al. 1981; Gustafsson & Pinter 1985). After ranking the motoneurones according to their current-threshold, the average threshold *difference* between successive S-motoneurones was smaller than that between successive FF-motoneurones (rat: 0.3 nA for S, 2.2 nA for FF; cat: 0.8 nA for S, 1.9 nA for FF; small steps significantly more common among S than among FF units, chi-square analysis, P<0.05).

The long-term matching perspective: Usage-dependent neuromuscular plasticity

It is well known that also during adult life the motoneurones determine, to a significant degree, the properties of their muscle units. Since the chronic stimulation experiments of Salmons & Vrbová (1969), it is known that many of these effects may be caused by long-term effects of motoneuronal activity patterns on muscle fibre properties. Thus, the fact that various aspects of motoneuronal activity are normally well adapted to contractile muscle unit properties (see Fig.2) leads naturally to the question of whether this matching is based on direct causal relationships, e.g. on long-term 'training effects' of motoneuronal discharge patterns on muscle unit properties. We have looked into this question using chronic electrical stimulation of muscle nerves to study the long-term effects of different activation patterns on muscle properties (for references, see Kernell & Eeerbeek 1989, 1991; Kernell 1992). The experiments were performed on ankle dorsiflexor muscles of the cat hindlimb (mainly peroneus longus). Chronic stimulation was given to the deafferented peroneal nerve (no pain or reflexes) in different patterns during 4-8 weeks. Thereafter the muscle properties were investigated in a final acute experiment. With respect to endurance these experiments showed that, irrespective of the pulse rate of stimulation (cf. Hudlická et al. 1982), activation during 5% of total time per day was sufficient for producing a marked increase of fatigue resistance (Burke-test) whereas 0.5% 'extra' activity left the muscle with a normal sensitivity to fatigue. These amounts of imposed daily activity are of interest in relation to published evidence that, at least in the rat, motoneurones that were likely to have fatigue-resistant muscle fibres were normally active more than 0.5% of total time per day (range 1.6-5.0%, for presumed FR motoneurones, Hennig & Lømo 1985; cf. also present symposium: Hensbergen & Kernell). In short, our results supported the general idea that, within a preset "adaptive range", long-term effects of motoneuronal activity are important for *contributing* to the normal kinds of endurance-related matching between muscle unit and motoneurone properties (for a more complete discussion, see Kernell & Eerbeek 1989; Kernell 1992).

During our chronic stimulation studies we also investigated how strict the linkage was between usage-evoked changes in fatigue-resistance and concurrent alterations in parameters that are commonly assumed to be closely related to neuromuscular endurance: (a) the electromyographic (EMG) behaviour during fatigue tests; and (b) the oxidative enzyme activity, as studied histochemically (staining for succinate dehydrogenase, SDH). Much to our surprise we found that the 0.5% and the 5% series of chronic stimulation, which gave markedly different effects on endurance, produced identical results with regard to both kinds of presumed fatigue correlate (Kernell et al. 1987). Furthermore, following a period of intense chronic stimulation, the rate of recovery toward normal properties was much slower for the EMG- than for the force-related behaviour during fatigue tests (Kernell & Eerbeek 1991). These findings are not meant to imply that EMG-changes and SDH-activities would be without any importance for fatigue-resistance in general. Our observations serve to underline, however, that it is still an open question which *types of fatigue* are critically dependent on EMG-associated parameters and/or on aspects related to the efficiency of oxidative metabolism.

References

Bawa P, Binder MD, Ruenzel P & Henneman E (1984). Recruitment order of motoneurons in stretch reflexes is highly correlated with their axonal conduction velocity. *Journal of Neurophysiology* **52**, 410-420.

Bigland-Ritchie B & Woods JJ (1984). Changes in muscle contractile properties and neural control during human muscular fatigue. *Muscle & Nerve* **7**, 691-699.

Botterman BR & Cope TC (1988). Motor-unit stimulation patterns during fatiguing contractions of constant tension. *Journal of Neurophysiology* **60**, 1198-1214.

Burke RE (1981). Motor units: anatomy, physiology and functional organization. In: *Handbook of Physiology - 1, vol.II, part 1*, Ed. Brooks VB, American Physiological Society, MD, pp.345-422.

Burke RE, Levine DN, Tsairis P & Zajac FE (1973). Physiological types and histochemical profiles in motor units of the cat gastrocnemius. *Journal of Physiology* **234**, 723-748.

Carp JS, Powers RK & Rymer WZ (1991). Alterations in motoneuron properties induced by acute dorsal spinal hemisection in the decerebrate cat. *Experimental Brain Research* **83**, 539-548.

Cope TC, Webb CB, Yee AK & Botterman BR (1991). Nonuniform fatigue characteristics of slow-twitch motor units activated at a fixed percentage of their maximum tetanic tension. *Journal of Neurophpysiology* **66**, 1483-1492.

Crow MT & Kushmerick MJ (1982). Chemical energetics of slow- and fast-twitch muscles of the mouse. *Journal of General Physiology* **79**, 147-166.

Emonet-Dénand F, Hunt CC, Petit J & Pollin B (1988). Proportion of fatigue-resistant motor units in hindlimb muscles of cat and their relation to axonal conduction velocity. *Journal of Physiology* **400**, 135-158.

Fleshman JW, Munson JB, Sypert GW & Friedman WA (1981). Rheobase, input resistance and motor-unit type in medial gastrocnemius motoneurons in the cat. *Journal of Neurophysiology* **46**, 1326-1338.

Garland SJ, Garner SH & McComas AJ (1988). Relationship between numbers and frequencies of stimuli in human muscle fatigue. *Jounal of Applied Physiology* **65**, 89-93.

Gustafsson B & Pinter MJ (1985). On factors determining orderly recruitment of motor units: a role for intrinsic membrane properties. *Trends in the Neurosciences* **8**, 431-433.

Henneman E & Mendell LM (1981). Functional organization of motoneuron pool and its inputs. In: *Handbook of Physiology - 1, vol.II, part 1*, Ed. Brooks VB, American Physiological Society, MD, pp.423-507.

Hennig R & Lømo T (1985). Firing patterns of motor units in normal rats. *Nature* **314**, 164-166.

Hudlická O, Tyler KR, Srihari T, Heilig A & Pette D (1982). The effect of different patterns of long-term stimulation on contractile properties and myosin light chains in rabbit fast muscles. *Pflügers Archiv* **393**, 164-170.

Jones DA, Bigland-Ritchie B & Edwards RHT (1979). Excitation frequency and muscle fatigue: Mechanical responses during voluntary and stimulated contractions. *Experimental Neurology* **64**, 401-413.

Kernell D (1966). Input resistance, electrical excitability, and size of ventral horn cells in cat spinal cord. *Science* **152**, 1637-1640.

Kernell D (1983). Functional properties of spinal motoneurons and gradation of muscle force. In: *Motor Control Mechanisms in Health and Disease*, Ed. Desmedt JE, Raven Press, New York, pp.213-226.

Kernell D (1986). Organization and properties of spinal motoneurones and motor units. *Progress in Brain Research* **64**, 21-30.

Kernell D (1992). Organized variability in the neuromuscular system: A survey of task-related adaptations. *Archives Italiennes de Biologie* **130**, 19-66.

Kernell D, Donselaar Y & Eerbeek O (1987). Effects of physiological amounts of high- and low-rate chronic stimulation on fast-twitch muscle of the cat hindlimb. II. Endurance-related properties. *Journal of Neurophysiology* **58**, 614-627.

Kernell D & Eerbeek O (1989). Physiological effects of different patterns of chronic stimulation on muscle properties. In: *Neuromuscular Stimulation. Basic Concepts and Clinical Implications*, Eds. Rose FC, Jones R & Vrbová G, Demos Publications, New York, pp.193-200.

Kernell D & Eerbeek O (1991). Recovery following intense chronic stimulation: A physiological study of cat's fast muscle. *Journal of Applied Physiology* **70**, 1763-1769.

Kernell D, Eerbeek O & Verhey BA (1983). Motor unit categorization on basis of contractile properties: an experimental analysis of the composition of the cat's m. peroneus longus. *Experimental Brain Research* **50**, 211-219.

Kernell D & Hultborn H (1990). Synaptic effects on recruitment gain: a mechanism of importance for the input-output relations of motoneurone pools? *Brain Research* **507**, 176-179.

Kernell D & Monster AW (1981). Threshold current for repetitive impulse firing in motoneurones innervating muscle fibres of different fatigue sensitivity in the cat. *Brain Research* **229**, 193-196.

Kernell D & Monster AW (1982a). Time course and properties of late adaptation in spinal motoneurones in the cat. *Experimental Brain Research* **46**, 191-196.

Kernell D & Monster AW (1982b). Motoneurone properties and motor fatigue. An intracellular study of gastrocnemius motoneurones of the cat. *Experimental Brain Research* **46**, 197-204.

Milner-Brown HS, Stein RB & Yemm R (1973). Changes in firing rate of human motor units during linearly changing voluntary contractions. *Journal of Physiology* **230**, 371-390.

Salmons S & Vrbová G (1969). The influence of activity on some contractile characteristics of mammalian fast and slow muscles. *Journal of Physiology* **201**, 535-549.

Thomas CK, Johansson RS & Bigland-Ritchie B (1991). Attempts to physiologically classify human thenar motor units. *Journal of Neurophysiology* **65**, 1501-1508.

Woods JJ, Furbush F & Bigland-Ritchie B (1987). Evidence for a fatigue-induced reflex inhibition of motoneuron firing rates. *Journal of Neurophysiology* **58**, 125-137.

Regulation of motorneuron firing rates in fatigue

B. R. Bigland-Ritchie

Quinnipiac College and John B. Pierce Laboratory, 290 Congress Avenue, New Haven, C.T. 06519, U. S. A.

Abstract. In 1980 we presented evidence suggesting that, during fatigue, motoneuron firing rates are regulated to match changes in muscle contractile speed. Here we describe more recent experiments designed to test that hypothesis, and to determine what physiological mechanisms may be involved. These include direct measurement of firing rate and contractile speed changes in fatigue from various types of exercise, and an ischemia test which showed that some input from the fatigued muscle must be involved. Other results do not support the suggestion that a decline in motoneuron firing rate is primarily due to reduced excitatory input from muscle spindles, or from inhibition from mechanoreceptors activated directly by slowing of contractile speed. Rather, they suggest that muscle metabolite accumulation is necessary, which probably excites Group III and IV afferent nerve endings, since firing rate changes were only seen when fatigue was induced by contractions which cause large changes in intramuscular metabolite composition (e.g. ischemia or sustained MVC). None were observed in fatigue from low force intermittent contractions in which all energy is derived aerobically. Our results also suggest that the factors responsible for initiating reflex inhibition may be the same as those which cause slowing of relaxation rates, thus ensuring that both parameters change in parallel. The functional consequences of such a mechanism are discussed.

In 1980, at the Ciba Foundation Symposium on human muscle fatigue we presented evidence suggesting that during a sustained maximal voluntary contraction motoneuron firing rates decline as fatigue develops. Despite this, however, the muscle can still remain fully activated by voluntary effort because the frequency required to elicit maximum force from a fatigued muscle declines in proportion to the slowing of muscle contractile speed. We speculated that adjustment of these rate changes may require some feedback mechanism from the muscle, but stated that "whether or not such a regulatory process actually exists remains to be determined". The present article describes subsequent work from this laboratory designed to determine the extent to which the central nervous system does indeed adjust its firing rates when muscle contractile speed is changed, and to elucidate what mechanisms must be involved.

Relation between motoneuron firing rates and muscle contractile speed

In animal experiments, the discharge rates recorded from nerves supplying slow muscles such as soleus are generally slower than those from nerves to muscles with faster contractile properties (e.g. gastrocnemius). But in such experiments it is seldom possible to estimate accurately the relative intensity of the contraction. Conversely, using conventional human EMG recording techniques during high-force voluntary contractions, it is generally not possible to discriminate potentials from individual motor units. This problem was overcome by the use of tungsten microelectrodes, which provide records with a high signal-to-noise ratio, and which allowed us to make the first accurate measurement of motoneuron discharge rates in maximal voluntary contractions (MVC). For the slow soleus muscle the upper limit of firing rates that can be elicited by voluntary effort was only 10.7 ± 2.9 Hz, compared to 31.1 ± 10.1 and 29.9 ± 8.6 Hz respectively for the faster biceps brachii and adductor pollicis muscles (Bellemare et al., 1983). These MVC firing rates were directly related to each muscle's twitch and/or tetanic contraction (CT) and half-relaxation (1/2RT) times. Similar measurements have since been made from other muscles.

When a MVC is sustained, the slowing of muscle contractile speed with fatigue is mainly evident as a prolongation of relaxation, with little change in contraction times (Fig 1A). We found that, as fatigue developed, motoneuron firing rates recorded from the adductor pollicis (AP) muscle decline in direct proportion to changes in 1/2RT (Bigland-Ritchie et al. 1983a&b). A similar firing rate decline with fatigue has since been measured in sustained MVCs of tibialis anterior (TA), first dorsal interosseous (FDI), quadriceps, soleus and biceps brachii (Kukulka et al, 1986; Woods et al., 1987; Vøllestad et al., 1988; Thomas et al., 1989; Bigland-Ritchie et al., 1992b). But because of the contractile slowing, this firing rate decline did not necessarily result in any loss of muscle activation (Fig 1A&B).

Muscle activation by voluntary effort.
The degree to which a muscle can be activated by the CNS in voluntary contractions can be demonstrated most directly by comparing its force output to that elicited by supramaximal tetanic stimulation of its motor nerve (Bigland-Ritchie, 1981); but this method is not always practical. In 1954 Merton showed that the degree of CNS muscle activation by voluntary efforts can also be assessed from the amplitude of twitches superimposed on the voluntary contraction in relation to that elicited from the relaxed muscle. When all motor units respond with maximum tetanic force no additional force can be elicited (Fig 1C&D). Subsequently Belanger & McComas (1981) developed this twitch occlusion or twitch interpolation technique more fully; and it is now widely used by various other groups. Indeed, Gandevia and McKenzie have used this technique in many studies on a wide range of muscles (e.g. McKenzie et al. 1992). By using double shocks, they find that failure to activate <1% MVC can be detected.

In the absence of fatigue, some people are able to achieve complete twitch occlusion on their first attempt. Others need practice, and still others never achieve complete twitch occlusion no matter how hard they try. In our experience mean control MVC muscle activation values for a group of well trained, highly motivated subjects, provided with both auditory and visual feedback, often range from 95-98%. However, as fatigue develops these high levels of muscle activation become increasingly difficult to achieve, particularly when the fatiguing exercise is of long duration. For example, almost full muscle activation can usually be retained during a 60 s sustained MVC in which the force declines by 30-50%, but may be reduced by 5-10% when the same force loss results from intermittent low force contractions repeated for 30 min.

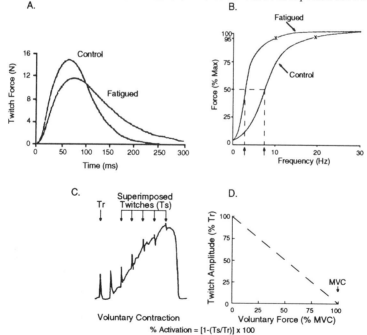

Fig 1. A & B. Twitches and force-frequency relations before and after contractile slowing. C. Occlusion of superimposed twitches as the voluntary force increases; and D the relation between them.

Functional Implications

Motor units are usually excited at 8-10 Hz when first recruited in voluntary contractions. Thus, they rarely, if ever, respond with single twitches, since at these rates some twitch fusion is already evident (Thomas et al., 1991). Nor are they often required to generate and sustain maximum tetanic force, except under laboratory conditions. Indeed, the capacity for prompt and sensitive force gradation requires that excitation rates be limited to those which elicit forces on the steep part of the force-frequency curve. But this frequency range shifts readily with changes of contractile speed. Thus, it seems mandatory for motor control that there must be some mechanism which regulates motoneuron firing rates in relation to changes in contractile speed.

The force or power output elicited from a muscle or motor unit by any given excitation rate depends on both the amplitude and duration of the underlying twitch properties, and hence the degree of fusion between twitch responses. Consequently, if twitch duration increases because of contractile slowing, as in fatigue, maximum force is generated at lower MN firing rates. Less well recognized is that when a fatigued muscle is excited at *submaximal* rates these may elicit a higher percentage of both the current and original maximum force; i.e. the relation between excitation rate and force output shifts toward lower rates. For example, an excitation rate which normally elicits about 10% maximal force may generate 50% of the now reduced maximal value after contractile slowing with fatigue (Fig 1B). Many other conditions commonly encountered in daily life, such as changes in muscle length and/or temperature, also change the relation between excitation rate and force output, mainly because they change muscle contractile speed. Thus, if a task requiring a constant force output is to be performed successfully under any of these conditions, firing rates must be appropriately adjusted. While motoneuron firing rates are largely determined by the time course of motoneuron after-hyperpolarization, which increases with activity (Kernell & Monster, 1982), it is unclear how this CNS process would necessarily be coordinated closely with changes of contractile speed in the peripheral muscle. Thus, it seems essential that the CNS be provided with some feedback originating from the fatigued muscle.

The difficulty in achieving 100% muscle activation by voluntary effort demonstrates that the CNS rarely drives motoneurons to fire at rates which exceed the minimum required for maximum force generation (Fig 1B). However, with contractile slowing, the rate needed to achieve maximum force declines so that, if firing rates remained unchanged, it would become easier to activate the muscle maximally by voluntary effort. However, this is never found in practice. All subjects find that the task of twitch occlusion gets progressively more difficult. Most studies report either no change or a reduction in MVC muscle activation with fatigue (e.g. Bigland-Ritchie, 1984; McKenzie et al. 1992). These observations in themselves provides strong evidence that firing rates are closely regulated; for motor control is, in fact, well maintained during different types of fatiguing exercise which cause a wide range of contractile speed changes.

Possible Mechanisms for regulating motoneuron firing rates during fatigue

Central Fatigue.

The firing rates of motoneurons are set initially by the strength of the excitatory input they receive and by differences between their biophysical properties. In a series of elegant studies Kernell and his colleagues (e.g. Kernell & Monster, 1982) showed that motoneuron after-hyperpolarization increases in response to prolonged constant current injection and causes a decline in firing rate similar to that seen in a sustained human MVC. Thus, it seemed reasonable to suppose that firing rate changes result from a reduced motoneuron responsiveness, despite a constant excitatory motor drive; i.e. central fatigue. However, it is hard to see how this mechanism alone would necessarily provide the accurate adjustment of firing rates to changes in contractile speed. Since changes in contractile speed may vary widely in different exercise conditions (see below) some sensory feed-back from the muscle seems to be required. We therefore attempted to separate the roles of possible central and peripheral mechanisms in the following way.

Ischemia Test for reflex involvement.
The test relied on the fact that local ischemia maintains a muscle in its fatigued state, with no recovery of either force or contractile speed, until its blood supply is restored. During a 40 s MVC executed with a blood pressure cuff inflated motoneuron firing rates declined in the usual way (Fig 2). No recovery of discharge rates was seen when the subject made a second 10 s MVC after 3 min rest with the local blood supply to the fatigued muscle still occluded. However, 3 min after the cuff was released MVC force and firing rates had both recovered fully. Thus 3 min is ample time for recovery of any changes in excitability of CNS neurons, and the depressed rates recorded in the second MVC must have resulted from some input from the fatigued muscle. Similar results were obtained when this protocol was applied to both adductor pollicis and quadriceps. We found also that these results could not be explained by either failure of neuromuscular transmission or an inability to activate the muscle fully under ischemic conditions (Woods et al.,1987).

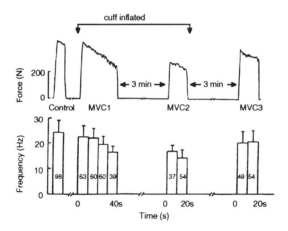

Fig 2. Test to determine whether motoneuron firing rates are influenced by afferent input from the fatigued muscle.

Nature of Afferent input

Possible muscle afferents which might serve to regulate motoneuron firing rates during fatigue include: 1) inhibition from mechanoreceptors responding directly to changes in muscle contractile speed; 2) the response of Group III & IV free nerve endings to changes in muscle metabolites; and 3) reduced motoneuron facilitation by muscle spindles consequent to fatigue of intrafusal fibers or reduced gamma drive.

Mechanoreceptors; temperature and length changes in the absence of fatigue.
The first possibility, that firing rate changes were due to input from receptors which monitor changes in muscle mechanical properties *per se*, was tested by measuring motoneuron firing rates when muscle contractile speed was altered in the absence of fatigue. For this purpose, we varied contractile speed in two ways: first, by changing muscle temperature; and second, by changing muscle length. Both conditions are frequently encountered in daily life, and require that accurate motor control be retained.
    When the FDI and AP muscles were cooled by 5°C (33-28°C) both CT and 1/2RT values increased; and these increases exceeded those observed following fatigue from a 60 s sustained MVC. Shortening the TA muscle from mid- to short-length shifted the force/frequency response (as in Fig 1B), such that the stimulus rate required to generate 50% maximum force increased by at least 5Hz; a change we could easily detect by spike recording. Yet neither procedure influenced the firing rates. There was no difference between the distribution of firing rates recorded during MVC contractions of FDI made at 28°C and 33°C (Bigland-Ritchie, 1992a). Similarly, no differences were found between the distribution of TA firing rates recorded at short and mid-muscle lengths during contractions of 50%, 75% or 100% MVC

(Bigland-Ritchie, 1992b). Thus, the afferent input arising during fatigue does not appear to respond directly to changes in the mechanical properties of the muscle. We found these results surprising since clearly motor control is in fact well maintained when muscles contract at different lengths, and wide swings of temperature are common, especially for hand muscles. Under these conditions some CNS knowledge of contractile speed changes would seem to be required.

Muscle spindle input.
Hagbarth and his colleagues (e.g. Bongiovanni & Hagbarth, 1990) suggest that the decline in firing rates with fatigue is not due to an inhibitory reflex, but rather to reduced facilitatory drive from muscle spindles. Amongst other evidence they find that firing rates in 1a afferents decline during a sustained voluntary contraction (Macefield et al., 1991). Macefield et al. (1992) also found that, if a muscle is deafferented by applying local anesthetic distal to the recording site, the firing rates recorded from motor axons by microneurography during maximum voluntary efforts are depressed compared to those in a MVC of intact muscle. This suggests that normal MVC firing rates cannot be achieved without motoneuron facilitation by muscle spindles. However, since the initial firing rates recorded after deafferentation were similar to those normally found only after fatigue, it is hard to conclude that deafferentation abolishes the normal reduction in motoneuron firing rate with fatigue. Nor can these results be attributed to removing the influence of any particular afferent type. Moreover, there is no test for effort maximallity when recording from a paralyzed muscle.

Inhibition via Group III & IV afferents responding to muscle metabolic changes.
It is well known that Group III & IV nerve endings can be excited by many of the metabolites which normally accumulate in, and may cause, fatigue (Kniffki et al,. 1981). They also have input to inhibitory interneurons in the spinal cord. Moreover, the decline in motoneuron firing rates is best demonstrated in sustained maximal or ischemic contractions where the muscle blood supply is necessarily occluded and changes in fatigue-related intramuscular metabolites are particularly great. In contrast, when the quadriceps muscle was fatigued by repeated low-force contractions in which the energy was supplied from aerobic sources, muscle biopsies showed no change in intramuscular metabolites during the first 30 min of exercise. In this case, since there was no depletion of energy substrates, the MVC force loss appeared to result from failure of excitation-contraction coupling (Vøllestad et al., 1988). We argued, therefore, that if inhibitory reflexes arise only in response to metabolic changes, little or no decline in motoneuron firing rates should occur during fatigue from this form of exercise.

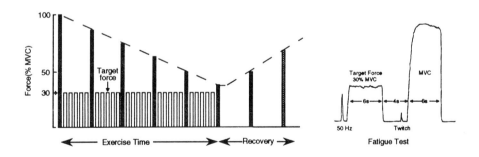

Fig 3. Schematic illustration of intermittent 30% MVC protocol and a fatigue test applied every 2 min.

The protocol used to test this hypothesis is shown in Fig 3. It consisted of 30% MVC isometric contractions of quadriceps each held for 6 s with 4 s rest periods between. In the previous study muscle biopsies taken after 5, 15 and 30 min showed no changes in metabolic composition. Every 2 min a "fatigue test" was performed consisting of a 6 s MVC with superimposed shocks, followed in the next rest period by either a brief burst of 50 Hz stimulation or a single (or double) shock (Fig 3B). Motoneuron firing rates were recorded during each test MVC, and during the subsequent 30% MVC target force contraction. Various parameters were measured for both twitch and tetanic responses to assess changes in muscle contractile speed. The exercise was continued until the MVC and responses to 50 Hz stimulation had declined by at least 40%. During this period we found that firing rates, recorded during both MVC or target force contractions, did not change significantly. Nor was there any slowing of contractile speed. When measured from tetanic responses, half-relaxation times remained unchanged throughout the exercise; but twitch CT and 1/2RT values both actually got significantly shorter (Rice et al., in preparation). Mean values for voluntary muscle activation gradually fell from 95% in control contractions to about 85% as MVC force declined. Curiously, despite the constant firing rates, the MVC integrated EMG declined. This might suggest either dropout of units after they had lost almost all capacity to generate force, or progressive failure of neuromuscular transmission (see Fuglevand et al., 1992).

Fatigue from intermittent 100% MVC contractions
Similar measurements were also made when fatigue was induced by 10 fully maximal quadriceps contractions, each again held for 6 s with 4 s rest between. However, in this case, alternate experiments were conducted with and without the muscle blood supply occluded by a cuff. Otherwise all measurements were similar to those for the intermittent 30% MVC contraction protocol.

When the circulation was occluded the changes with time in all values (force, IEMG, motoneuron firing rates, contractile speed, etc.) were essentially similar to those in a 60 s sustained MVC (Bigland-Ritchie et al 1983 a,b). When the circulation was intact, so that accumulated metabolites were removed between contractions, the rate of change of all parameters was reduced. The MVC and 50 Hz forces declined by only about 20 %, and motoneuron firing rates showed no change through the ninth contraction; but some slowing of muscle contractile speed was evident. Unlike those in the 30% MVC contractions, the EMG values increased progressively throughout the protocol. Thus, motoneuron firing rates, contractile speed and other fatigue-related parameters can, to some extent, change independently (Rice et al., 1992).

General comments

1. *The nature of fatigue.* Research in this area has always been hampered by confusion as to the most appropriate definition of "fatigue". For example, fatigue is often defined as "an inability to maintain the required or expected force" (see Stuart, this volume). Whereas for our purposes we define it as "any reduction in the force-generating capacity (measured as the MVC), regardless of the task performed" (Bigland-Ritchie & Woods, 1984). Clearly, when the task is to generate only 30% MVC, the first definition would claim that no fatigue occurred, despite up to 50% decline in MVC force. Indeed, by definition, a given submaximal force has now become maximal whenever it can no longer be maintained. In other situations other definitions may also be required. For example in dynamic exercise, where fatigue may best be expressed as the decline in power output which need not necessarily be closely correlated with force (see Jones; and also Sargeant; this volume).

2. *Variability of fatigue related events.* Another common misconception is that fatigue-related changes in the muscle and CNS follow a common pattern, regardless of how the fatigue is generated. However, when different types of exercise are used to reduce MVC force by a given amount, the changes of contractile speed and motoneuron firing rates are quite different in each case. For isometric contractions, slowing of contractile speed is most pronounced in a sustained MVC; but no slowing was seen in tetanic responses during low-force intermittent contractions. Indeed, CT and 1/2RT values measured from twitches actually got significantly shorter. Similarly, motoneuron firing rates may decline by 40% in a MVC sustained for only 60 s or not change at all in 30 min of low-force intermittent contractions, despite the same force reduction in each case. However, the functionally essential close correlation between firing rate and contractile speed changes is generally well preserved. This close correlation could be achieved if the same metabolic events which slow relaxation during fatigue also trigger the reflex which inhibits motoneuron firing rates.

We have found only one situation, fatigue from intermittent 100% MVCs, where motoneuron firing rates and contractile speed appear to vary independently. Relaxation rates got slightly but consistently slower while firing rates remained almost unchanged. Contractile slowing with fatigue, which is most evident in the relaxation phase (Bigland-Ritchie et al., 1983), is thought to be due to the increase in H^+ and Pi (Cady et al, 1989). Perhaps the threshold level at which they start to affect relaxation is lower than that needed to trigger reflex inhibition. However, when the same contractions were executed under ischemic conditions both relaxation and firing rates declined as in a sustained MVC.

3. *Reflex regulation*. The experiments described here, together with those from several other laboratories, leave little doubt that motoneuron firing rates decline in high-force contractions which occlude the blood supply. Furthermore, the reduced firing rates do not necessarily reduce muscle activation, since fusion frequencies become lower when muscle contractile speed gets slower. But the mechanisms whereby firing rates are regulated to match changes in muscle contractile speed remain unknown. While various processes have been proposed, the notion that fatigue-related metabolite accumulation initiates an inhibitory reflex is strongly supported by our recent finding that the usual decline in motoneuron firing rates was absent when fatigue was caused by exercise in which no muscle metabolites accumulate, despite up to 50% reduction in MVC force. In contrast, the decline in firing rates is most evident in fatigue from sustained MVCs, or during intermittent contractions with blood supply occluded where metabolites accumulation is maximal. Thus, reflex inhibition appears to be triggered by some metabolic event; and it is probably mediated by group III and IV muscle afferents which are known to be excited by various fatigue-associated metabolic events (Kniffki et al., 1981). The role of changes in motoneuron after-hyperpolarization and/or withdrawal of their facilitation by spindles is unlikely to be great; for otherwise these would still induce <u>some</u> motoneuron firing rate decline even when the influence of input from group III & IV afferents has been removed. Furthermore, if inhibitory reflexes are elicited only by changes in muscle metabolic composition, it is clear why firing rates did not change when contractile speed was slowed by cooling or increased muscle length in the absence of fatigue.

4. *Advantages in minimizing firing rates*. There are important functional advantages in keeping motoneuron firing rates as low as possible in voluntary contractions. First, this preserves motor control, since force regulation is most sensitive when motoneuron firing rates are limited to the steep part of the force-frequency curve, and would be severely compromised if MVC firing rates exceeded the minimum required to elicit a fully fused tetanus. At supratetanic rates no additional force is generated, but the contraction becomes less efficient because of the extra energy associated with the Ca^{++} turnover per impulse. Low firing rates also protect the integrity of e/c coupling and neuromuscular transmission (Bigland-Ritchie et al, 1979 & 1984).

When a muscle is stimulated continuously at rates above 10-20 Hz the amplitude of the evoked M-wave declines at a rate directly related to the stimulus frequency. (It can also be restored by reducing the rate). However, we have never been convinced that transmission was impaired in fatigue of <u>voluntary</u> contractions studied in a wide range of muscles when fatigued in a variety of ways (Bigland-Ritchie et al, 1979 & 1982; cf Bellemare & Garzaniti, 1988; Fuglevand et al, 1992). The amplitudes and areas of M-waves evoked by single shocks to the motor nerve usually remain constant or increase, despite up to 50% force decline, even in MVCs of TA extended for up to 5 min (Thomas et al, 1989), during 3 min of post fatigue ischemic rest (Woods et al, 1987), and during fatigue from intermittent submaximal contractions of adductor pollicis and diaphragm continued for 30-50 min (Bellemare & Bigland-Ritchie, 1987). In the few cases where M-wave amplitudes declined somewhat (sustained MVC of FDI) this was offset by a greater increase in M-wave duration with no change in area indicating dispersion between potentials from different units, rather than transmission block. Similarly low excitation rates also preserve the integrity of e/c coupling (Jones et al, 1979; Westerblad et al, 1991). Preserving the robust integrity of e/c coupling and neuromuscular transmission would be unlikely in the absence of inhibitory reflexes. Indeed, in exercise of long duration, there is evidence of some breakdown in these processes (see above; Vøllestadet al., 1988; Fuglevand et al., 1992).

A reduction in firing rate serves to optimize force during fatigue, but only if there is a corresponding slowing of contractile speed to increase twitch fusion. Otherwise the reduced rates must inevitably limit the degree to which the muscle can be activated by voluntary effort. Thus it makes excellent sense that where no contractile slowing accompanies fatigue (e.g. during 30% MVC intermittent contractions) inhibitory reflexes are absent. Thus it is intuitively appealing to suggest that both are driven by the same metabolic events.

Problems.

The arguments presented here were selected to support the hypothesis that motoneuron firing rates are regulated during fatigue in relation to changes of muscle contractile speed; and also that this relies mainly on inhibitory reflexes triggered by metabolic changes in the muscle. However, the identity of the particular metabolites is not known. While it is attractive to suggest that common compounds influence both relaxation and firing rates, any substance which stimulates group III & IV free nerve endings must penetrate the sarcolemma with the required time course.

Many other fatigue-related observations also remain difficult to explain. For example, the firing rates of individual motor units often decline with time even when the force exerted is extremely low. Under these conditions it is hard to believe that sufficient metabolites accumulate to initiate either contractile slowing or reflex activity when only a few units may be active; and other mechanisms such as after-hyperpolarization may be responsible. Clearly there must be other purely CNS mechanisms which can be called on when needed. For example, force regulation is well maintained when muscle contractile speed is altered by changes in muscle length or temperature. But it is not clear how this is done since these procedures did not effect motoneuron firing rates in our experiments, presumably because no accumulation of metabolites was involved.

Acknowledgments: I am grateful for the major contributions to this work made by the many colleagues with whom I have been privileged to work; and for assistance from Dr. C. L. Rice and Mr. R. N. Kieft in preparing the manuscript. The work was supported by USPHS grants NS14756 & HL 30026, and by fellowships from the Muscular Dystrophy Associations of US and Canada.

References

Belanger AY, & McComas AJ (1981). Extent of motor unit activation during effort. *Journal of Applied Physiology* **50**, 538-544.

Bellemare F & Bigland-Ritchie B (1987). Central components of diaphragmatic fatigue assessed from bilateral phrenic nerve stimulation. *Journal of Applied Physiology* **62**, 1307-1316.

Bellemare F & Garzaniti N (1988). Failure of neuromuscular propagation during human maximal voluntary contraction. *Journal of Applied Physiology* **64**, 1084-1093.

Bellemare F, Woods JJ, Johansson R, (1983). Motor unit discharge rates in maximal voluntary contractions of three human muscles. *Journal of Neurophysiology* **50**, 1380-1392.

Bigland-Ritchie B (1981) EMG and fatigue of human voluntary contractions. In Ciba Foundation Symposium 82 "Human muscle fatigue: physiological mechanisms" Ed. Porter and Whelan. Pitman Medical. London. pp. 130-156.

Bigland-Ritchie B & Woods JJ (1984) Changes in muscle contractile properties and neutral control during human muscular fatigue. Invited reviews: in *Muscle and Nerve*. **7**, 691-699.

Bigland-Ritchie B, Jones DA, & Woods JJ (1979). Excitation frequency and muscle fatigue: Electrical responses during human voluntary and stimulated contractions. *Experimental Neurology* **64**, 414-427.

Bigland-Ritchie B, Kukulka CG, Lippold OCJ & Woods JJ. (1981). The absence of neuromuscular transmission failure in sustained maximal voluntary contractions. *Journal of Physiology (London)* **330**, 265-278.

Bigland-Ritchie B, Johansson R, Lippold OCJ and Woods JJ. (1983). Contractile speed and EMG changes during fatigue of sustained maximal voluntary contractions. *Journal of Neurophysiology* **50** (**1**), 313-324.

Bigland-Ritchie B, Johansson R, Lippold OCJ, Smith, S and Woods JJ. (1983). Changes in motoneurone firing rates during sustained maximal voluntary contractions. *Journal of Physiology* **340**, 335-346.

Bigland-Ritchie B, Thomas CK, Rice CL, Howarth JV, & Woods JJ (1992a). Muscle temperature, contractile speed, & motoneuron firing rates during human voluntary contractions. *Journal of Applied Physiology* (Submitted)

Bigland-Ritchie B, Furbush F, Gandevia SC, & Thomas CK (1992b). Voluntary discharge frequencies of human motoneurons at different muscle lengths. *Muscle & Nerve* **15** (**2**), 130-136.

Bongiovanni LG, & Hagbarth K-E (1990). Tonic vibration reflexes elicited during fatigue from maximal voluntary contractions in man. *Journal of Physiology* **423**, 1-14.

Cady EB, Elshove H, Jones DA, & Moll A (1989). The metabolic causes of slow relaxation in fatigued human skeletal muscle. *Journal of Physiology* **418**, 327-337.

Fuglevand AJ, Zackowski KM, Huey KA, & Enoka RM (1992). Impairment of neuromuscular propagation during human fatiguing contractions at submaximal forces. *Journal of Physiology* (In Press).

Jones DA, Bigland-Ritchie B, & Edwards RHT (1979) Excitation frequency & muscle fatigue: Mechanical responses during voluntary & stimulated contractions. *Experimental Neurology* **64**, 414-427.

Kernell D (1984). The meaning of discharge rate: Excitation-to-frequency transduction as studied in spinal motoneurones. *Archives Italiennes de Biologie* **122**, 5-15.

Kernell D, & Monster AW (1982). Time course and properties of late adaptation in spinal motoneurones of the cat. *Experimental Brain Research* **46**, 191-196.

Kniffki K-D, Mense S & Schmidt (1981). Muscle receptors with fine afferent fibers which may evoke circulatory reflexes. *Circulation Research* **48**, 125-131.

Macefield G, Hagbarth KE, Gorman R, Gandevia SC & Burke D (1991). Decline in spindle support to alpha - motoneurons during sustained voluntary contractions. *Journal of Physiology* **440**, 497-512.

Macefield G, Gandevia SC, Bigland-Ritchie B, Gorman R & Burke D, (1992). The discharge rate of human motoneurones innervating ankle dorsiflexors in the absence of muscle afferent feedback. *Journal of Physiology* (in press).

McKenzie DK, Bigland-Ritchie B, Gorman RB, & Gandevia SC. (1992). Central and peripheral fatigue of human diaphragm and limb muscles assessed by twitch interpolation. *Journal of Physiology (London)* (In Press).

Merton, P. A. (1954) Voluntary strength and fatigue. *Journal of Physiology (London)*. **128**, 553-564.

Rice CL, Vøllestad NK & Bigland-Ritchie B (1992). Dissociation of fatigue-related neuromuscular events. *Medicine and Science in Sports and Exercise* (In press).

Thomas C K, Woods JJ, & Bigland-Ritchie B (1989). Neuromuscular transmission and muscle activation in prolonged maximal voluntary contractions of human hand and limb muscles. *Journal of Applied Physiology* **67**, 1835-1842.

Thomas C K, Bigland-Ritchie B & Johansson, RS (1991). Force-frequency relations of human thenar motor units. *Journal of Neurophysiology* **65** (**6**), 1509-1516.

Vøllestad NK, Sejersted OM, Bahr R, Woods JJ, & Bigland-Ritchie B (1988). Motor drive and metabolic responses during repeated submaximal voluntary contractions in man. *Journal of Applied Physiology* **64**, 1421-1427.

Westerblad H, Lee JA, Lannergren J & Allen DG. (1991). Cellular mechanisms of fatigue in skeletal muscle. *American Journal of Physiology* **261** (**30**), C195-C209.

Woods JJ, Furbush F, & Bigland-Ritchie B (1987). Evidence for a Fatigue-Induced Reflex Inhibition of Motoneuron Firing Rates. *Journal of Neurophysiology* **58**, 125-136.

Central and peripheral components to human isometric muscle fatigue

S.C. Gandevia

Department of Clinical Neurophysiology, Institute of Neurological Sciences, The Prince Henry Hospital and Prince of Wales Medical Research Institute, University of New South Wales, Sydney, Australia

Abstract During isometric exercise with limb muscles the maximal voluntary force declines. This is accompanied by a decline not only in the peripheral force generating capacity of the muscle but also by a progressive impairment in the voluntary capacity to generate optimal force from the muscle as assessed by twitch interpolation. There is a reduction in motor unit discharge rate during maximal static contractions. Several mechanisms contribute to this including reflex inhibition from small-diameter afferents and dysfacilitation from muscle spindle endings. Central neuronal mechanisms are critical in maintaining the highest force output from muscles during fatigue.

Fatigue produced in isometric electrically-stimulated contractions provides a tool to examine changes in the peripheral force generating capacity. This technique ensures complete electrical activation of the muscle fibres and avoids the metabolic and mechanical complexities associated with concentric and eccentric contractions: events occurring proximal to the neuromuscular junction are inevitably eliminated. If one investigates maximal voluntary isometric contractions, there are immediate advantages and disadvantages. First, the motoneurones are under voluntary control and their discharge patterns are those occurring naturally rather than those imposed artificially (synchronous activity in all motor units, usually at a fixed frequency). This advantage is important because motoneurone discharge rates decline in sustained maximal isometric contractions in a range of muscles (e.g. Bigland-Ritchie et al. 1983, 1986; Bellemare et al. 1983; Kukulka et al. 1986; Gandevia et al. 1990a). This appears to optimize force production because the contractile spreed of the muscle declines also. Indeed, the improvement in sustaining force with an appropriately controlled decline in frequency has been observed with tetanic stimulation of several human muscles (quadriceps femoris, Bigland-Ritchie et al. 1979; extensor digitorum brevis, Grimby et al. 1981; adductor pollicis, Marsden et al. 1983). Furthermore, force may be initiated more efficiently by inclusion of "doublet" discharges (e.g. Burke et al. 1976; Zajac & Young 1980), and fatigue may be diminished by using slightly irregular rather than regular discharge patterns (Bevan et al. 1992). However, reliance on the central nervous system to drive the motoneurones introduces its own limitations. Afferent feedback from the contracting muscles and nearby skin and joints can exert short- and long-latency reflex effects on the motoneurone pool and affect the continual central planning for the contraction. In addition, although a sustained maximal isometric effort is being attempted, it is possible (indeed likely, see below) that the drive reaching the motoneurone pool is often less than optimal for force production. However, this limitation provides insight into the properties of so-called "central" fatigue.

In what follows I discuss several aspects of control of motoneurone discharge during maximal isometric contractions of both fresh and fatigued muscles. These include use of the twitch interpolation method to document suboptimal levels of motoneuronal drive and the possible mechanisms responsible for the decline in discharge of motoneurones during sustained contractions.

Terms

The term 'maximal effort' will refer to an attempted maximal contraction under isometric conditions in which the subject receives continuous verbal and auditory feedback of performance. 'Muscle fatigue' refers to any exercise-induced reduction in the force-generating capacity of the muscle in a maximal effort as assessed by sensitive forms of twitch interpolation. 'Voluntary activation' denotes the degree of activation of the test (stimulated) muscles assessed by twitch interpolation, while 'central fatigue' refers to a progressive decrease in the level of voluntary activation during sustained or repetitive effort.

Twitch interpolation reveals suboptimal maximal efforts

Does the central nervous system drive the motoneurones to optimal frequencies during maximal voluntary efforts and, if so, is this activity continued when the voluntary efforts are repeated in the presence of overt peripheral fatigue? This question addresses an upper limit to human motor performance. A lower limit of performance, the ability to produce voluntarily a single discharge in the lowest threshold motor units without feedback has been established, at least for distal hand muscles (see Gandevia & Rothwell 1987).

The first studies to examine these questions physiologically compared the peak force achieved with tetanic stimulation of the nerve innervating an intrinsic hand muscle with the maximal force produced voluntarily: these forces matched well (Merton, 1954; Bigland & Lippold 1954). Regrettably, there are few nerve-muscle combinations in which this can be examined. Stimulation of a single nerve rarely produces all the force in one direction at a joint and, for large proximal muscles, it may be uncomfortable. Maximal voluntary efforts also encourage 'trick' movements involving synergists and remote stabilizing muscles not innervated by the stimulated nerve. An alternative is to interpolate a stimulus to a nerve trunk or intramuscular nerve fibres during a maximal voluntary effort such that additional force evoked by the stimulus at the appropriate latency indicates a deficiency in recruitment, and/or firing frequency of motoneurones. Application of this method to adductor pollicis revealed that voluntary activation was complete in fresh muscle and muscle fatigued under ischaemia (Merton 1954). This view has been supported by Bigland-Ritchie and colleagues when assessing maximal voluntary discharge rates during isometric efforts (e.g. Bigland-Ritchie et al. 1983, 1992; Bellemare et al. 1983). However, Belanger and McComas (1981) sounded a note of caution when reporting that ankle plantar-flexor muscles appeared more difficult to activate fully, a finding for soleus which is well known to electromyographers.

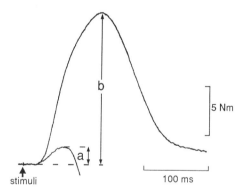

Figure 1. A representative control twitch produced by paired stimuli (10 ms apart) to the elbow flexors. Superimposed on it is the response to the same supramaximal stimuli during an attempted maximal voluntary effort. Voluntary activation of the stimulated muscles is calculated by subtraction of the ratio b/a from 1, expressed as a percentage.

Our studies initially highlighted subjects' ability to drive some limb muscles (abductor digiti minimi, tibialis anterior and biceps brachii/brachialis) and the diaphragm fully during brief efforts when given feedback (Gandevia & McKenzie 1985, 1988a,b; Gandevia et al. 1990b). This occurred when we applied sensitive methods to examine the small force increments added by the interpolated stimuli (Hales & Gandevia 1988) and averaged optimal trials. However, on many occasions subjects did not quite voluntarily activate the muscle fully as indicated by the small force increments (superimposed twitches) produced by supramaximal stimuli (Figs. 1 and 2). Such increments were usually less than 10% of the resting control twitch amplitude

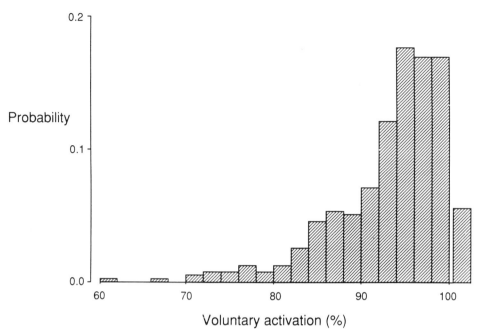

Figure 2. A histogram of the voluntary activation achieved by 20 subjects during 20 maximal voluntary isometric efforts of elbow flexors in the absence of fatigue. Flexors innervated by both the musculocutaneous and radial nerves were stimulated.

indicating that volition achieved more than 90% of the stimulated muscle group's force.

We have recently examined this formally for biceps brachii/brachialis when healthy subjects made 20 brief maximal isometric contractions of the elbow flexors (at 90°) and comparable contractions of the inspiratory muscles at functional residual capacity. Fatigue was eliminated by leaving a 1-2 min interval between efforts. All subjects received equal practice. For the elbow flexors, interpolated stimuli were delivered simultaneously to biceps, brachialis and brachioradialis, and for the diaphragm, stimuli were delivered to both phrenic nerves via wire electrodes in the neck. Subjects varied significantly in their ability to activate each muscle. Apparent extinction of the twitch occurred in only a small percentage of 'maximal' efforts (Fig. 2). Voluntary activation of the diaphragm was significantly lower for the diaphragm than elbow flexors (Allen et al. 1992). This trend, previously noted in a smaller group of subjects (McKenzie et al. 1992), emerged whether all contractions or only the better ones from each subject were analysed.

Three aspects of these results are notable. First, it is overgenerous to assume that well-motivated, healthy subjects routinely generate the optimal output from a fresh limb muscle. Thus, the discharge frequency of some high-threshold motor units must be critically placed along their force-frequency relationships, or some motor units are not recruited in this static phase of the contraction, or both. Second, voluntary activation is not necessarily similar for different motoneurone pools. This is expected given the greater corticofugal excitation to distal than proximal and truncal muscles revealed by a variety of clinical and electrophysiological techniques (e.g. Hughlings Jackson 1865; Leyton & Sherrington 1917; Phillips & Porter 1977; Rothwell et al. 1987; Bohannon & Smith 1987; Colebatch & Gandevia 1988). However, any reflexes operating during maximal efforts do not eliminate this variability in descending motor drive between different muscles. The correlation between voluntary activation assessed with twitch interpolation and descending motor "command" has been emphasized elsewhere (Gandevia, 1992).

When maximal isometric contractions are repeated over a range of duty cycles from 5-50%, there is a progressive decline in voluntary activation (McKenzie & Gandevia 1991). This is accompanied by a more marked reduction in the amplitude of the twitch responses. Contractile speed did not decline with the lowest duty cycles, but was prominent with a duty cycle of 50%. Progressive difficulty in maintenance of full voluntary activation was noted by Thomas et al.

(1989) in single prolonged contractions. During repeated submaximal isometric contractions with elbow flexors over 45 min punctuated by maximal efforts, voluntary drive declines progressively in a group of subjects (Lloyd et al. 1991; see Fig. 3). The probability of achieving optimal output from the muscles declined as the exercise proceeded. This trend is evident under a range of isometric exercise protocols and must be considered the normal responses to this type of exercise.

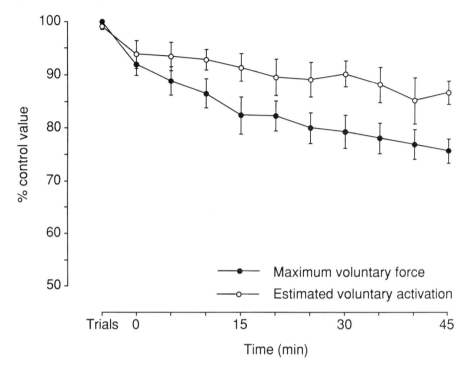

Figure 3. Maximal voluntary force of elbow flexors during submaximal isometric exercise (30% maximal force, 6 s contractions with 4 s rest intervals) in 13 healthy subjects. While maximal force (and twitch forces - not shown) declined over 45 min of exercise, there was also a decline in voluntary activation of biceps brachii and brachialis. This was assessed with paired stimuli (10 ms interval). This decline was statistically significant for the population of subjects and many individuals. Further details are contained in Lloyd et al. (1991) from which this data has been modified.

Changes in motoneurone discharge rate during fatigue

During a sustained isometric contraction of an intrinsic hand muscle Marsden et al. (1969) found that the discharge rate declined progressively. Bigland-Ritchie and colleagues studied this phenomenon for a range of limb muscles including adductor pollicis, biceps brachii, quadriceps and tibialis anterior (e.g. Bellemare et al. 1983; Bigland-Ritchie et al. 1992). The decline in motoneurone rate appeared to parallel the decline in half-relaxation of the stimulated muscle such that it seemed possible to activate the muscle fully in a maximal effort despite the decline in motoneurone discharge rate (Bigland-Ritchie et al. 1983). Such a matching between contractile properties and motoneurone discharge rate is intrinsically appealing, although it is now clear that many mechanisms contribute to it.

Reflex inhibition of the motoneurone pool may arise due to increased activity in small-diameter afferents within the contracting muscle. Thus, the decline in maximal motoneurone discharge rates (and force production) persists as long as the contracting muscles are held ischaemic with a sphygmomanometer cuff inflated above systolic pressure (Bigland-Ritchie et al. 1986; Woods et al. 1987). Intrinsic motoneurone properties which could have translated a constant excitatory drive into an adapting discharge (e.g. Kernell, 1965; Kernell & Monster 1982) would presumably recover despite the arterial occlusion. However, adaptation of discharge frequency obtained with current injection into the motoneuronal soma may not mimic the effect of constant post-synaptic excitation (Spielman et al. 1991). Further evidence in favour of reflex inhibition as a mediator of the phenomenon was obtained by finding that voluntary activation (assessed electromyographically) of ankle dorsiflexor muscles was impaired following electrically-induced fatiguing contractions produced under ischaemic conditions (Garland et al. 1988), an impairment not substantially affected by a pressure block of large-diameter axons (Garland 1991). Given that the afferent fibres and central neural machinary exist for a reflex inhibition of motoneurones elicited by ischaemic contractions (see also Hayward et al. 1988), this mechanism must contribute to the decline in motoneurone discharge.

A second phenomenon which could contribute to the decline in motoneurone discharge rate is a reduction in the discharge frequency of muscle spindle endings. In simple isometric contractions in human subjects, the fusimotor system is recruited producing an increase in discharge of most spindle endings within the contracting muscle (e.g. Vallbo 1974; Burke 1981). Such discharges should facilitate the motoneurone pool via mono- and oligo-synaptic spinal reflexes along with long-latency, partly transcortical reflexes. Hagbarth and colleagues have argued that a reduction in spindle discharge and hence of motoneuronal facilitation (i.e. dysfacilitation) would contribute to the reduction in motoneuronal discharge frequency (e.g. Bongiovanni & Hagbarth, 1990). Microneurographic recordings from muscle spindle afferents support this view (Macefield et al. 1991b). Subjects held force constant for 60 s with ankle dorsiflexors in the range of 30-60% maximal voluntary force. Peak spindle discharge frequency occurred during the ramp up to the target force and then the frequency declined rapidly in the next few seconds and then more slowly. The absolute decline was more pronounced for spindle afferents with a higher mean discharge rate and when several contractions had been performed. These changes in spindle discharge, particularly the initial decline are evident in earlier published recordings of spindle behaviour, but their significance has not been emphasized until recently. Importantly, this finding indicates that the fusimotor-muscle spindle system does not effectively compensate for contractile fatigue: electromyographic activity rose during the constant-force contractions, yet the spindle discharge declined. As indicated elsewhere, many factors could lead to the decline in spindle discharge ranging from a reflex reduction or adaptation in the discharge of fusimotor neurones, to intrafusal fatigue (see Macefield et al. 1991b). Recent studies have focused on the discharge of fusimotor axons during short and long ischaemic contractions in the cat (Anastasijevic et al. 1987; Ljubisavljevic et al. 1992). During electrical stimulation of the muscle nerve or ventral roots, fusimotor discharge to triceps surae displayed a late increase (at 60-120 s). This appeared to be related to a reflex input from the limb arising during muscle ischaemia, presumably from group III and IV afferents. However, any increase in fusimotor discharge in sustained contractions by intact human subjects fails to overide other factors causing spindle discharge to decline.

Another approach to examine the changes in nett reflex excitation during maximal voluntary contractions has been to record the discharge of single motor axons destined for a particular muscle when the muscle is completely paralysed by a nerve block distal to the recording electrode. Under such circumstances the subject wills a maximal effort of the muscle while the motor axon discharge is recorded microneurographically. Any input from the contracting muscle (and similarly innervated synergists) is unable to reach the central nervous system because of the distal local anaesthetic block. For motor axons innervating tibialis anterior and ulnar-innervated intrinsic hand muscles, the discharge frequency during attempted maximal voluntary efforts of the paralysed muscles is lower (by about a third) than when muscle afferent feedback is present (Gandevia et al. 1990a; Macefield et al. 1991a). This suggests that a nett facilitation arises from reflex inputs (presumably muscle spindle afferents) during maximal static efforts of 30-60 s duration. Motoneurone frequency failed to adapt significantly after the first 5 s during the deafferented contractions indicating that reflex inputs mediate the decline in discharge when muscles are normally innervated. Some data for the ulnar motor axons are shown in Fig. 4. The decline in motoneurone rate in the first few seconds may reflect spindle dysfacilitation but the later decline will also reflect the inhibition from small diameter fibres.

The concepts developed above depend upon a somewhat simplistic notion of the "excitability" of the motoneurone pools in which muscle spindle endings provide facilitation and group III and IV afferents inhibition. Even at a spinal level the synaptic circuitry involved in mediating such overall effects is complex (e.g. McCrea 1992). For example, no mention has been made of pre-synaptic inhibition of primary muscle spindle afferents and other inputs to the motoneurone pool. Presynaptic inhibition of group Ia afferents can be modulated by descending motor commands, being significantly reduced at the onset of a ramp contraction of ankle plantar flexors (Meunieur & Pierrot-Deseilligny 1989). It returns towards control levels during the attainment of the target force and imposes constraints on motoneurone excitability and discharge frequency. Also, group Ib autogenetic inhibition will be modulated during sustained voluntary contractions (Fournier et al. 1983), and it is also subject to presynaptic inhibition. Thus, while Golgi tendon organs continue to respond to dynamic force changes during partially fused tetani in the cat, the inhibitory post-synaptic potentials which they induce in the motoneurone diminish rapidly (Zytnicki et al. 1990) due to presynaptic inhibition (Lafleur et al. 1992).

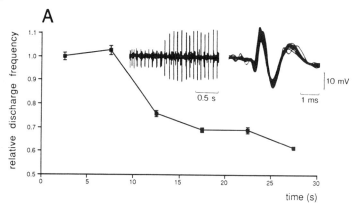

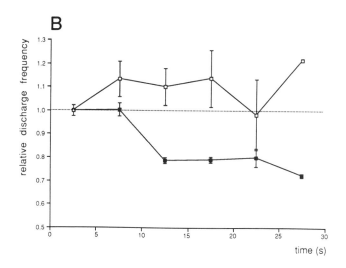

Figure 4. *A*, sequential analysis of motor unit discharge frequencies during maximal voluntary efforts of 20-30 s duration; data from 4 subjects expressed in relative terms (mean ±SE). Spike trains recorded from motor units were analysed in 5 s epochs. Note the decline in motor unit discharge frequencies 10-15 s after the commencement of a maximal voluntary contraction. *Inset*, motor unit spike train recorded from first dorsal interosseous 15 s after the commencement of a maximal voluntary contraction. During its passage through the contracting muscle the microelectrode approached a large amplitude motor unit; this particular spike train consisted of 27 impulses, the superimposed action potentials are illustrated on the right. *B*, sequential analysis of the motor axon (open symbols) and motor unit (closed symbols) (1 subject). There was no progressive decline in discharge frequency of the deafferented motor axons.

Finally, given that individual muscles can be used differently during a variety of motor tasks, it is likely that reflexes acting on the motoneurone pool will behave differently - so called task-depedence. This is clearly evident for group Ia excitatory effects on the soleus motoneurone pool during walking and running (e.g. Capaday & Stein, 1987), but must also occur during isometric tasks. The diaphragm, the crucial inspiratory muscle, can be driven fully during maximal static inspiratory and also expulsive efforts (Gandevia & McKenzie 1985; Gandevia et al. 1990b), yet it is only in the latter type of effort (which elevates abdominal pressure and threatens diaphragm perfusion) that marked central fatigue develops (Gandevia et al. 1992). Regulation of motoneuronal excitability and hence of maximal motor unit discharge rate will be task dependent. This aspect of central motor control remains to be further investigated.

References

Allen GM, McKenzie DK & Gandevia SC (1992). Differences in voluntary activation of the human diaphragm and elbow flexors during attempted maximal efforts. *Proceedings of the Australian Physiological and Pharmacological Society* **23**, 23P.

Anastasijevic R, Jocic M & Vuco J (1987). Discharge rate and reflex responses of fusimotor neurons during muscle ischaemia. *Ezperimental Neurology* **97**, 340-344.

Belanger AY & McComas AJ (1981). Extent of motor unit activation during effort. *Journal of Applied Physiology* **51**, 1131-1135.

Bellemare F, Woods JJ, Johansson RS & Bigland-Ritchie B (1983). Motor unit discharge rates in maximal voluntary contractions of three human muscles. *Journal of Neurophysiology* **50**, 1380-1392.

Bevan L, Laouris Y, Reinking RM & Stuart DG (1992). The effect of the stimulation pattern on the fatigue of single motor units. *Journal of Physiology (London)*, in press.

Bigland-Ritchie B, Dawson NH, Johansson RS & Lippold OCJ (1986). Reflex origin for the slowing of motoneurone firing rates in fatigue in human voluntary contractions. *Journal of Physiology (London)* **379**, 451-459.

Bigland-Ritchie B, Furbush F, Gandevia SC & Thomas CK (1992). Voluntary discharge frequencies of human motoneurons at different muscle lengths. *Muscle & Nerve* **15**, 130-137.

Bigland-Ritchie B, Johansson RS, Lippold OCJ & Woods JJ (1983). Contractile speed and EMG changes during fatigue of sustained maximal voluntary contractions. *Journal of Neurophysiology* **50**, 313-324.

Bigland-Ritchie B, Jones DA & Woods JJ (1979). Excitation frequency and muscle fatigue: electrical responses during human voluntary and stimulated contractions. *Experimental Neurology* **64**, 414-427.

Bigland B & Lippold OCJ (1954). Motor unit activity in the voluntary contractions of human muscle. *Journal of Physiology (London)* **125**, 322-335.

Bohannon RW & Smith MB (1987). Assessment of strength deficits in eight paretic upper extremity muscle groups of stroke patients with hemiplegia. *Physical Therapy* **67**, 522-25.

Bongiovanni LG & Hagbarth K-E (1990). Tonic vibration reflexes elicited during fatigue from maximal voluntary contractions in man. *Journal of Physiology (London)* **423**, 1-15.

Burke D (1981). The activity of human muscle spindle endings in normal motor behavior. In *International Review of Physiology, Volume 25, Neurophysiology IV*. Ed, Porter R. University Park Press. Baltimore. pp.91-126.

Burke RE, Rudomin P & Zajac FE (1976). The effect of activation history on tension production by individual muscle units. *Brain Research* **109**, 515-529.

Capaday C & Stein RB (1987). Difference in the amplitude of the human soleus H reflex during walking and running. *Journal of Physiology (London)* **392**, 513-522.

Colebatch JG & Gandevia SC (1989). The distribution of muscular weakness in upper motor neuron lesions affecting the arm. *Brain* **112**, 749-763.

Fournier E, Katz R & Pierrot-Deseilligny E (1983). Descending control of reflex pathways in the production of voluntary isolated movements in man. *Brain Research* **288**, 357-377.

Gandevia SC (1992). Cortical output, strength, and muscle fatigue. In: *Science and Practice in Clinical Neurology: Reviews in Pathophysiology, Diagnosis and Management*. Eds, Gandevia SC, Burke D & Anthony M. Cambridge University Press, Cambridge, in press.

Gandevia SC, Macefield G, Burke D & McKenzie DK (1990a). Voluntary activation of human motor axons in the absence of muscle afferent feedback. *Brain* **113**, 1563-1581.

Gandevia SC & McKenzie DK (1985). Activation of the human diaphragm during maximal static efforts. *Journal of Physiology (London)* **367**, 45-56.

Gandevia SC & McKenzie DK (1988a). Human diaphragmatic endurance during different maximal respiratory efforts. *Journal of Physiology (London)* **395**, 625-638.

Gandevia SC & McKenzie DK (1988b). Activation of human muscles at short muscle lengths during maximal static efforts. *Journal of Physiology (London)* **407**, 599-613.

Gandevia SC, McKenzie DK & Plassman BL (1990b). Activation of human respiratory muscles during different voluntary manoeuvres. *Journal of Physiology (London)* **428**, 387-403.

Gandevia SC & Rothwell JC (1987) Knowledge of motor commands and the recruitment of human motoneurons. *Brain* **110**, 1117-1130.

Garland SJ (1991). Role of small diameter afferents in reflex inhibition during human muscle fatigue. *Journal of Physiology (London* **435**, 547-558.

Garland SJ, Garner SH & McComas AJ. (1988). Reduced voluntary electromyographic activity after fatiguing stimulation of human muscle. *Journal of Physiology (London)* **401**, 547-556.

Grimby L, Hannerz J & Hedman B (1981). The fatigue and voluntary discharge properties of single motor units in man *Journal of Physiology (London)* **316**, 545-554.

Hales JP & Gandevia SC (1988). Assessment of maximal voluntary contraction with twitch interpolation: an instrument to measure twitch responses. *Journal of Neuroscience Methods* **25**, 97-102.

Hayward L, Breitbach D & Rymer Z (1988). Increased inhibitory effects on close synergists during muscle fatigue in the decerebrate cat. *Brain Research* **440**, 199-203.

Jackson JH (1865). Lectures on hemiplegia. *Clinical Lectures and Reports by the Medical and Surgical Staff of the London Hospital* **2**, 297-332.

Kernell D (1965). The adaptation and the relation between discharge frequency and current strength of cat lumbosacral otoneurons stimulated by long-lasting injected currents. *Acta Physiologica Scandinavica* **65**, 65-73.

Kernell D & Monster AW (1982). Time course and properties of late adaptation in spinal motoneurones of the cat. *Experimental Brain Research* **46**, 191-196.

Kukulka CG, Russell AG & Moore MA (1986). Electrical and mechanical changes in human soleus muscle during sustained maximum isometric contractions. *Brain Research* **362**, 47-54.

Lafleur J, Zytnicki D, Horcholle-Bossavit G & Jami L (1992). Depolarization of Ib afferent axons in the cat spinal cord during homonymous muscle contraction. *Journal of Physiology (London)* **445**, 345-354.

Leyton AS & Sherrington CS (1917). Observations on the excitable cortex of the chimpanzee, orang-utan and gorilla. *Quarterly Journal of Experimental Physiology* **11**, 135-222.

Ljubisavljevic M, Jovanovic K & Anastasijevic R (1992). Changes in discharge rate of fusimotor neurones provoked by fatiguing contractions of cat triceps surae muscles. *Journal of Physiology (London)* **445**, 499-513.

Lloyd AR, Gandevia SC & Hales JP (1991). Muscle performance, voluntary activation, twitch properties and perceived effort in normal subjects and patients with chronic fatigue syndrome. *Brain* **144**, 85-98.

Macefield G, Gandevia SC, Bigland-Ritchie B, Gorman R & Burke D (1991a). The discharge rate of human motoneurones innervating ankle dorsiflexors in the absence of muscle afferent feedback. *Journal of Physiology (London)* **438**, 219P.

Macefield G, Hagbarth K-E, Gorman R, Gandevia SC & Burke D (1991b). Decline in spindle support to α-motoneurones during sustained voluntary contractions. *Journal of Physiology (London)* **440**, 497-512.

McCrea D (1992). Can sense be made of spinal interneuron circuits? *Behavioral Brain Sciences*, in press.

McKenzie, DK, Bigland-Ritchie B, Gorman RB & Gandevia SC (1992). Central and peripheral fatigue of human diaphragm and limb muscles assessed by twitch interpolation. *Journal of Physiology (London)*, in press.

McKenzie DK & Gandevia SC (1991). Recovery from fatigue of human diaphragm and limb muscles. *Respiration Physiology* **84**, 49-60.

Marsden CD, Meadows JC & Merton PA (1969). Muscular wisdom. *Journal of Physiology (London)* **200**, 15P.

Marsden CD, Meadows JC & Merton PA (1983). "Muscular wisdom" that minimizes fatigue during prolonged effort in man: peak rates of motoneuron discharge and slowing of discharge during fatigue. In: *Advances in Neurology: Motor Control Mechanisms - Health and Disease*. Ed, Desmedt J. Raven Press. New York. pp 169-211.

Meunier S & Pierrot-Deseilligny E (1989). Gating of the afferent volley of the monosynaptic stretch reflex during movement in man. *Journal of Physiology (London)* **419**, 753-763.

Merton PA (1954). Voluntary strength and fatigue. *Journal of Physiology (London)* **123**, 553-564.

Phillips CG & Porter R (1977). *Corticospinal Neurones*. Academic Press. London.

Rothwell JC, Thompson PD, Day BL, Dick JPR, Kachi T, Cowan JMA & Marsden CD (1987). Motor cortex stimulation in intact man. *Brain* **110**, 1173-1190.

Spielmann JM, Laouris Y, Nordstrom MA, Reinking RM & Stuart DG (1991). The relation between motor-neuron adaptation and muscle fatigue. *Third IBRO World Congress of Neuroscience*, Montreal, Canada. pp. 470.

Thomas CK, Woods JJ & Bigland-Ritchie B (1989). Impulse propagation and muscle activation in long maximal voluntary contractions. *Journal of Applied Physiology* **67**, 1835-1842.

Vallbo AB (1974). Human muscle spindle discharge during isometric voluntary contractions. Amplitude relations between spindle frequency and torque. *Acta Physiologica Scandinavica* **90**, 319-336.

Vøllestad NK, Sejersted OM, Bahr R, Woods JJ & Bigland-Ritchie B (1988). Motor drive and metabolic responses during repeated submaximal contractions in humans. *Journal of Applied Physiology* **64**, 1421-1427.

Woods J, Furbush F & Bigland-Ritchie B (1987). Evidence for a fatigue-induced reflex inhibition of motoneuron firing rates. *Journal of Neurophysiology* **58**, 125-137.

Zajac FE & Young JL (1980). Properties of stimulus trains producing maximum tension-time area per pulse from single motor units in medial gastrocnemius muscle of the cat. *Journal of Neurophysiology* **43**, 1206-1220.

Zytnicki D, Lafleur J, Horcholle-Bossavit, G, Lamy F & Jami L (1990). Reduction of Ib autogenetic inhibition in motoneurons during contractions of an ankle extensor muscle in the cat. *Journal of Neurophysiology* **64**, 1380-1389.

Change of α motoneurone excitability during fatigue by voluntary contraction

J. Duchateau and K. Hainaut

Laboratory of Biology, Université Libre de Bruxelles, 28, av. P. Héger, CP 168, 1050 Brussels, Belgium

It has been reported in a previous paper that the amplitude of the short and medium latency reflex components recorded in response to a sudden stretch in the human first dorsal interosseous are reduced after fatigue by voluntary contraction (Balestra et al. 1992). These changes can be the result of: (1) reduced spindle output (Macefield et al. 1991) and/or (2) decreased excitability of α motoneurones (MN) through inhibitory muscle afferences (Woods et al. 1987; Garland and Mc Comas 1990). The present study was designed to obtain further informations on the mechanisms whereby reflex activities are impaired during fatigue.

Experimental methods

Ten healthy subjects (9 males and 1 female) ranging between 24 and 44 years old took part to this investigation. The Hoffmann reflex (HR) was recorded during voluntary contractions (10-15% of MVC) of the thenar muscles by using the method introduced by Deuschl et al.(1985). This method consists of the electrical stimulation of the median nerve at the wrist with a stimulus strength set near the threshold response of the motor fibres. The electromyogram (EMG) of the abductor pollicis brevis was recorded by means of surface electrodes in a belly-tendon fashion. The signal was amplified (1000x), filtered (10-5000 Hz), rectified and averaged (64 sweeps). In order to exclude peripheral neuromuscular alterations due to fatigue in the interpretation of the results, the HR amplitude was normalized as a function of the maximal M wave amplitude and also as a percentage increment above the basal level of EMG activity. Muscle fatigue was induced by a sustained MVC which was interrupted when the force was reduced to 50% of its maximal value. To avoid any recovery of the EMG activity during the post-fatigue recording, a cuff placed around the arm was inflated (250 mmHg) just before the end of the fatigue test.

Results

In control condition, the mean ($\pm$ SD, n = 10) latency and duration of HR are 29.6 $\pm$ 1.6 ms and 11.0 $\pm$ 1.3 ms respectively. After the fatiguing contraction (mean duration : 101 $\pm$ 16.1s), the duration of HR is significantly increased by 21.2 $\pm$ 14.2% (P < 0.005) whereas its latency is not statistically modified. HR amplitude is found to be drastically reduced by 51.3 $\pm$ 13.2% of the control value. When HR amplitude is normalized as a function of the M waves amplitude or of the basal EMG activity, its value is significantly (P < 0.005) reduced to 69.8 $\pm$ 21.3% and 71.8 $\pm$ 13.2% respectively. These changes persist as long as the cuff is inflated but return to control values within 5 min after the ischemic block is interrupted.

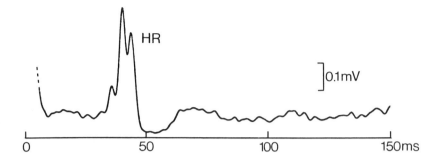

Figure 1. Typical example of an HR response in one subject.

Discussion

The main finding of this work is that the amplitude of HR is drastically reduced after fatigue by MVC. After normalization of the reflex amplitude, in order to avoid changes of peripheral neuromuscular alterations due to fatigue in the interpretation of the results, a significant deficit of about 30% persist which can only be related to decreased α MN excitability. This observation of a depressed excitability of the α MN pool after fatigue is in line with the recent results obtained by Garland and McComas (1990) on the soleus after electrically evoked fatigue tests. In the present study, the magnitude of the reflex inhibition is very similar to that recorded for the short latency stretch reflex after a comparable fatigue test (Balestra et al, 1992). Although this comparison is made in two different hand muscles, it suggests that spindle fatigue should not be the prime cause of the stretch reflex decrease after fatigue but that most of the reduction can be explain by inhibition of the α MN pool.

References

Balestra C, Duchateau J & Hainaut K (1992). Effects of fatigue on the stretch reflex in a human muscle. Electroencephalography and Clinical Neurophysiology **85**, 46-52.

Deuschl G, Schenk E & Lücking CH (1985). Long-latency responses in human thenar muscles mediated by fast conducting muscle and cutaneous afferents. Neuroscience Letters **55**, 361-366.

Garland SG & Mc Comas AJ (1990). Reflex inhibition of human soleus muscle during fatigue. Journal of Physiology **429**, 17-27.

Macefield G, Hagbarth KE, Gorman R, Gandevia SC & Burke D (1991). Decline in spindle support to α-motoneurones during sustained voluntary contractions. Journal of Physiology **440**, 497-512.

Woods J, Furbush F & Bigland-Ritchie (1987). Evidence for a fatigue-induced reflex inhibition motoneurone firing rates. Journal of Neurophysiology **58**, 125-137.

Fatigue-related impairment of neural drive to muscle

A. J. Fuglevand and R. M. Enoka

Department of Exercise & Sport Sciences, University of Arizona, Tucson, AZ 85721 USA

The amplitude of the surface-detected electromyogram (EMG) increases during sustained, submaximal isometric contractions. This increase in EMG is due to an increase in motor unit recruitment and discharge rate that is necessary to maintain a target force in the presence of a declining force capacity of the contractile machinery. We have found, however, that the eventual inability to maintain force at a target level is due in part to an inadequate level of neural drive to muscle.

Evidence for impaired neural drive

We recently examined changes in evoked (M wave) and voluntary EMG signals associated with sustained contractions at different submaximal force levels (Fuglevand et al., 1992). Thirty-two subjects were assigned to one of three groups which differed as to the target force of the fatigue task: 20, 35, or 65% of the maximum voluntary contraction (MVC) force. The fatigue task involved a sustained isometric abduction of the index finger at the target force. Abduction force and first dorsal interosseus EMG were monitored throughout the task, which was terminated when the force dropped below 90% of the target for more than 2 seconds. M waves were elicited prior to and immediately after the fatigue task. The rectified average EMG, the mean frequency of the EMG power spectrum, and the average force were determined for each 10% epoch of the fatigue task.

The average endurance times for the 20, 35, and 65% target force groups were 534 s, 246 s, and 66 s, respectively. The mean power frequency declined in parallel during the fatigue task for all three groups and reached a similar endpoint value (50, 43, and 45% of the initial value for the 20, 35, and 65% MVC groups, respectively) suggesting that metabolite-induced changes in the propagation velocity of muscle fiber action potentials were similar for the three groups. The amplitude of the voluntary EMG increased from 19.3 to 45.2% of the pre-fatigue MVC value for the 20% MVC group, from 31.5 to 54.5% for the 35% MVC group, and from 59.6 to 81.4% for the 65% MVC group (Fig. 1). Voluntary EMG, therefore, failed to reach maximum levels (pre-fatigue MVC) during the fatigue task for any of the three force groups.

The fatigue task also caused a significant depression of M-wave amplitude for all three groups; immediately after the fatigue test, M-wave amplitude was 76.2, 73.6, and 88.3% of pre-fatigue amplitude for the 20, 35, and 65% MVC groups. The decline in M-wave ampli-

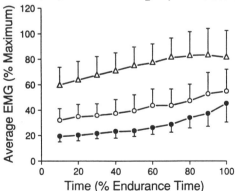

Figure 1. Mean (SD) changes in voluntary EMG amplitude during sustained isometric contractions at 20 % (•), 35% (o), and 65% (Δ) of MVC force (from Fuglevand et al., 1992).

tude, which reflects neuromuscular-propagation impairment, was greatest for the low-target force conditions. In a separate set of experiments involving nine subjects, the EMG from MVCs performed immediately after the fatigue task were diminished relative to pre-fatigue levels (61.9, 65.3, and 71.0% of pre-fatigue MVC for the 20, 35, and 65% MVC groups).

Potential mechanisms contributing to impaired neural drive

The fatigue-related deficit in voluntary EMG probably represents the net effect of at least six processes that limit the neural excitation of muscle (Fig. 2). These include: decreased excitatory input to motor neurons from the motor cortex (Maton, 1991) and muscle spindle afferents (Macefield et al., 1991); increased inhibitory input to motor neurons from metabolite-sensitive muscle receptors (Bigland-Ritchie et al., 1986) and Renshaw cells (McNabb et al., 1987); a reduction in motor neuron excitability (Kernell & Monster, 1982); and impaired neuromuscular propagation (Fuglevand et al., 1992). We suggest that impaired neural drive to muscle during sustained contractions contributes significantly to the decreased force capacity of the neuromuscular system.

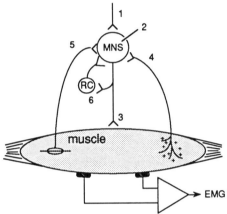

Figure 2. Processes that may interact to impair neural drive to muscle, as reflected in the surface EMG, during sustained contractions. 1) decrease in excitatory input from motor cortex 2) adaptation in motor neuron (MN) excitability 3) impairment of neuromuscular propagation 4) inhibition from metabolite-sensitive receptors 5) decrease in muscle spindle feedback 6) increased recurrent inhibition via Renshaw cells (RC).

References

Bigland-Ritchie B, Dawson NJ, Johansson RS & Lippold OCJ (1986). Reflex origin for the slowing of motoneurone firing rates in fatigue of human voluntary contractions. *Journal of Physiology* **379**, 451-459.

Fuglevand AJ, Zackowski KM, Huey KA & Enoka RM (1992). Impairment of neuromuscular propagation during human fatiguing contractions at submaximal forces. *Journal of Physiology,* in press.

Kernell D & Monster AW (1982). Motoneurone properties and motor fatigue: an intracellular study of gastrocnemius motoneurones of the cat. *Experimental Brain Research* **46**, 197-204.

Macefield G, Hagbarth K-E, Gorman R, Gandevia SC & Burke D (1991). Decline in spindle support to α-motoneurones during sustained voluntary contractions. *Journal of Physiology* **440**, 497-512.

Maton B (1991). Central nervous system changes in fatigue induced by local work. In: Atlan G, Beliveau L, Bouissou P (eds.), *Muscle fatigue. Biochemical and physiological aspects,* pp. 207-221. Paris: Masson.

McNabb N, Frank JS & Green HJ (1988). Recurrent inhibition during sustained contractions in humans. *Society for Neuroscience Abstracts* **14**, 948.

Afferent and spinal reflex aspects of muscle fatigue: Issues and Speculations

Douglas G. Stuart and Robert J. Callister

Department of Physiology, College of Medicine, University of Arizona, Tucson, Arizona 85724, USA.

"...during fatigue, motoneurone firing rates may be regulated by a peripheral reflex originating in response to fatigue-induced changes in the muscle..." (Bigland Ritchie et al. 1986)

Abstract In this article, the above quote from the work of Bigland-Ritchie and her colleagues is discussed in relation to afferent and spinal reflex mechanisms that could conceivably contribute to the reflex. The argument is first advanced that evaluation of this hypothesis should not be limited to studies on humans and other mammalian species. Rather, it should be extended to include invertebrates and other vertebrate groups, because it is likely that the neuromuscular mechanisms that reduce and delay muscle fatigue in glycolytic muscle cells have been subject to evolutionary conservation. Next, we address a concern of Bigland-Ritchie et al. (1986) that a controlled reduction in motoneurone firing rates during fatigue is attributable in part to the cells' intrinsic (biophysical) properties. We consider this possibility less likely than the operation of a more complex control strategy in which CNS-induced changes in the biophysical properties of motoneurones serve, themselves, to delay and reduce fatigue. In regard to the afferent and spinal reflex aspects of the Bigland-Ritchie hypothesis, we have argued that no single afferent species is dominant in the effects of afferent feedback on motoneurone discharge during fatiguing muscle contractions, at least before the onset of pain. Rather, as with reflex control of sustained and intermittent movements in the fresh (unfatigued) state, it is likely that *all* the limb afferents contribute, in a context-dependent fashion. Finally, it is proposed that the role of limb afferent input during fatigue should not be limited to consideration of restricted (private, specialized) spinal pathways. Instead, since at least the proprioceptive component of this sensory input has multifaceted responsibilities in motor control, all such responsibilities should be examined in the face of muscle fatigue.

The study of muscle fatigue (hereafter termed fatigue) can provide a framework for new perspectives on the operation of the motor control system, at both segmental and suprasegmental levels. For work at the segmental level, the topic of this article, it is sufficient to define fatigue as a "... failure to maintain the required or expected force" (Edwards 1981; for suprasegmental considerations, see Enoka & Stuart 1992). The segmental motor system is a term used to describe the integrated (systems) operation of brainstem/spinal motor circuitry, motor units, muscle receptors, and the segmental actions of muscle, joint and cutaneous afferents (reviewed in Binder & Mendell 1990). As reviewed elsewhere (Stuart & Enoka 1990), the systems approach to the segmental motor system has been dominated for thirty years by three areas of study: 1) the role of spinal interneurons in integrating descending command and sensory-feedback signals for the elaboration of spinal reflexes; 2) the mechanisms underlying the interneuronal pattern generation required for the execution of relatively stereotyped movements like breathing, chewing, swimming and walking; and 3) the phenomenon of orderly motor unit recruitment and its potential underlying mechanisms, such as Henneman's size principle. Now, a fourth area of study seems fruitful: testing ideas pertaining to muscle fatigue, such as the idea of Bigland-Ritchie et al. (1986) that is quoted above. It is argued below that the testing of their *sensory-feedback hypothesis* in a wide variety of animal species has important implications for furthering the understanding of the segmental motor system.

Evolutionary and phylogenetic considerations

To this point, the study of segmental aspects of fatigue has been limited almost exclusively to studies undertaken on mammalian species; notably cat, rat and human. However, the appearance of fatigue and the neural strategies employed to reduce and delay it are as ubiquitous in the animal kingdom as movement itself. Furthermore, the ability to cope with fatigue, even in a transitory fashion, is fundamental to the survival of all species. Hence, neural, neuromuscular, and muscular mechanisms of fatigue must surely be as subject to *evolutionary conservation* as other molecular, cellular and intercellular (systems) mechanisms that are fundamental to survival.

This need for *interphyletic awareness* (cf. Stuart 1985) in the study of fatigue is also supported by the proposition that the neurobiological aspects of muscle fatigue largely involve consideration of interactions between the CNS and glycolytic, rapidly-fatiguing muscle cells. The fatigue literature suggests that it is these cells on which the CNS and peripheral neuromuscular mechanisms can exert the most fatigue-reducing/delaying effect, whereas the eventual fatigability of oxidative, fatigue-resistant muscle cells is determined primarily by metabolic processes within the active muscle cells. Similarly, the presence or absence of temperature regulatory mechanisms (which primarily affect the rates of chemical and physical processes, rather than underlying mechanisms) and blood flow are not crucial for anaerobic metabolism during fatiguing contractions, but become critical factors when considering aerobic mechanisms during fatigue. This *neural vs. metabolic* division of fatigue mechanisms has presumably also been subject to the same evolutionary conservation that has resulted in a division of labor between the anaerobic *vs.* aerobic types of muscle fiber so prominent in both invertebrates (e.g., arthropods; Rathmayer & Maier 1987), which evolved in the Cambrian Period (approx. 570 million years ago) and non-mammalian vertebrates (e.g., lampreys, elasmobranchs and teleost fishes; Ogata 1988, Rome et al. 1988), which likewise appear very early in the fossil record. These points are emphasized first in this article, because investigations of motor control (including fatigue) in mammals can continue to derive much inspiration from considering the neural mechanisms and strategies that nature found so useful many millions of years ago, well before the appearance of mammalian species (e.g., Callister et al. 1992). Interestingly, while this viewpoint is now well accepted for molecular (e.g., genes, ion channels, myosin isoforms, Ca^{2+} binding proteins) and cellular (e.g., mitosis, metabolic pathways, synaptic transmission) mechanisms, it is less well appreciated at the systems and organismic levels of inquiry except perhaps in the study of the neural control of locomotion. In this area, the work of Grillner and colleagues on the lamprey (reviewed in Grillner et al. 1988, 1991) has provided new openings in the study of mammalian locomotion. Similarly, new insights into the control of multi-jointed movement have been provided by the study of the wiping reflex in frogs (Giszter et al. 1989; Ostry et al. 1991).

Muscle wisdom and the sensory-feedback hypothesis

As fatigue proceeds in conscious humans during both maximum voluntary contractions (MVCs) and imposed contractions of a selected pattern, there is a decrease in the rate of whole-muscle relaxation which lowers fusion frequency. This occurs concomitantly with a reduction in the rate of motoneurone discharge (e.g.: Dietz 1978; Marsden et al. 1976, 1983; Bigland-Ritchie et al. 1986). This association between force, relaxation and discharge rates is referred to as muscle wisdom. It should ensure that the CNS drive to fatiguing muscle does not exceed that necessary to produce the required force, and as such should serve to reduce and delay "central" fatigue within the CNS (cf. Enoka & Stuart 1992).

While the findings to date are particularly interesting, several features of muscle wisdom now require systematic investigation. For example: 1) several observations in the Marsden et al. (1983) report are puzzling (e.g., the EMG data in their Fig. 6) and require confirmation and extension; 2) similarly, an observation of Bigland-Ritchie et al. (1983; their Fig. 4B) is possibly at odds with a subsequent one of Binder-Macleod and McDermond (1992; their Figs. 1-4; cf. also Botterman & Cope 1988, and Cooper et al. 1988); 3) the boundary conditions of muscle wisdom remain relatively unexplored, such as comparison of repetitive *vs.* sustained contractions (e.g.: Duchateau & Hainaut 1985; Bergstrom & Hultman 1988), fatigue brought on by low- *vs.* high-frequency contractions (cf. Garland et al. 1988), short- *vs.* long-duration

Afferent and spinal reflex aspects of muscle fatigue

contractions (Bergstrom & Hultman 1988), and by different patterns of activation, including those of variable duty cycle (cf. Gandevia 1990; McKenzie & Gandevia 1991) and interpulse interval (Binder-Macleod & Barker 1991; Bevan et al. 1992; Laouris & Stuart, this volume); and 5) the relation of muscle wisdom to motor-unit type is relatively unexplored. However, indirect evidence suggesting that slow-twitch units may be less effected than fast-twitch ones (Dubose et al. 1987; Gordon et al. 1990) is in keeping with the evolutionary and phylogenetic considerations emphasized above. This latter evidence reinforces the need to test for the manifestation of muscle wisdom during fatiguing muscle contractions in a variety of animal species, in order to test the appealing notion that this strategy, too, has been subject to evolutionary conservation.

To account for muscle wisdom, Bigland-Ritchie and her colleagues have proposed the sensory-feedback hypothesis under consideration in this article. This hypothesis must coexist with orderly motor-unit recruitment and Henneman's size principle (for review: Binder & Mendell 1990) and, like the latter (Stuart & Enoka 1983), Bigland-Ritchie's hypothesis is simple to comprehend, it provides a unified means of viewing previous, present and future studies, and it is testable with present-day techniques in a variety of animal species.

Sensory feedback vs. motoneurone adaptation

In the same report in which Bigland Ritchie et al. (1986) advanced the sensory-feedback hypothesis, they cautioned that "...the decline in motoneurone firing rates seen during fatigue of a sustained maximum voluntary contraction may result primarily from changes in central motoneurone excitability; the time course of frequency changes are quite similar to that reported by Kernell and colleagues for changes in the discharge rates of cat single motoneurones in response to constant current injection (...Kernell & Monster 1982 a,b)". This caveat was prompted by the authors' recognition of the similarity in the on-average magnitude of the drop in firing rate (approx. 33 to 18 Hz) of motor units in their human subjects during a 40 second MVC and that (approx. 29 to 16 Hz) over the same time period during sustained intracellular stimulation of motoneurones in deeply anesthetized cats (e.g., compare Fig. 4A-B in Bigland-Ritchie et al. 1983 to Fig. 5 in Kernell & Monster 1982b). In this comparison, the adaptation reported by Kernell and Monster (1982a,b) is termed *late*: it occurs after the first 1-2 s of sustained stimulation in contrast to the more rapid drop in firing rate, termed *initial*, that occurs at the onset of stimulation. Our group (Spielmann et al. 1991) has considered these firing-rate declines in relation to evidence on: initial *vs.* late adaptation following sustained stimulation and *within-train vs. between-train* adaptation following intermittent stimulation (Llinás & Lopez-Barneo 1988; Spielmann et al. 1990; Spielmann 1991; Nordstrom et al. 1991); the neuropharmacology of after-hyperpolarization (e.g., Zhang & Krnjevic 1987; Hounsgaard et al. 1988) and; after-hyperpolarization under near passive and active (fictive locomotion) conditions (Brownstone et al. 1992). Collectively these results suggest: 1) similarities between initial and within-train, and late and between-train adaptation; 2) the obligatory nature of initial and late adaptation (but probably involving different mechanisms) in the presence of motoneurone after-hyperpolarization; 3) the mutability of motoneurone after-hyperpolarization (and hence initial and late adaptation), as effected by descending command signals, CNS state (e.g., passive *vs.* active) and associated transmitters and neuromodulators. On this basis, we believe it is premature to assume that after-hyperpolarization and its obligatory initial and late adaptation are features of motoneurone discharge during natural movements, such as during an MVC. Rather, it seems more attractive to test the possibility that the intrinsic (biophysical) properties are subject to an extrinsic (synaptically mediated) control by the CNS. Such a control mechanism could be context (task) dependent and serve to reduce and delay fatigue, at least on a temporary basis. It would seem that the intrinsic *vs.* extrinsic control of after-hyperpolarization (and hence intitial and late adaptation) is an important issue that must be resolved in parallel with consideration of the evidence (vide infra) that implicates sensory feedback in reducing motoneurone firing during fatiguing contractions.

Sensory-feedback vs. "interneuronal wisdom"

In a sense, the concept of muscle wisdom is an extension to dynamic (muscle activation) conditions of the now well-accepted principle that the morphological, biochemical, biophysical and physiological properties of spinal motoneurones are related in an interdependent manner to those of the muscle cells they innervate. Evidence for these interdependencies and the testing of additional ones are described in the literature on the size principle (e.g., Binder & Mendell

1990; Gardiner & Kernell 1990), nerve-to-muscle trophism in reduced animal preparations (Vrbová 1989) and muscle-to-nerve trophism (e.g., Czeh et al. 1978). In simple, but intuitively attractive language, the notion is now well accepted that motoneurones have an **a priori** knowledge about the force developing potential of the muscle cells they innervate. Of at least equal importance is a newly emerging literature which suggests that spinal interneurones have a similar **a prioi** knowledge about the mechanical properties of an entire limb when performing a task that involves more than one joint (e.g., Gielen et al. 1988; Gurfinkel et al. 1988; Koshland et al. 1991; Lacquaniti et al. 1991). This point is introduced here to emphasize that a thorough testing of the sensory-feedback hypothesis will not only require consideration of interactions between sensory-feedback during fatiguing contractions and the intrinsic (biophysical) *vs.* extrinsic (synaptically mediated) properties of motoneurones, but also between this feedback and populations of spinal interneurones that may respond to fatigue-induced sensory input in a fashion appropriate for the biomechanics of the entire limb.

Issues concerning sensory afferents and their central actions
Indirect evidence, derived from experiments on conscious humans using a variety of imaginative protocols, has implicated small diameter group III-IV afferents, presumably signaling changes in the metabolic status of muscle cells, in a reflex inhibition of motoneurones during fatigue (Bigland-Ritchie et al. 1986; Woods et al. 1987; Garland et al. 1988; Gandevia et al. 1990; Garland & McComas 1990; Garland 1991; Macefield et al. 1992; cf. Kulkulka et al. 1986). Direct evidence from reduced animal experiments supporting this logically appealing notion is limited and somewhat contradictory. While it is firmly established that muscle contraction reflexly increases cardiovascular and ventilatory function via group III-IV muscle afferent input (reviewed in Kniffki et al. 1981), the identity of the contraction-induced stimuli responsible for the increased activity in these small diameter afferents was unknown until recently. Now, however, their is evidence to suggest that known products of muscle metabolism (e.g., K^+, H^+ and arachadonic acid) can increase the discharge rates of some group III-IV afferents (Kaufmann et al. 1988; Rotto & Kaufmann 1988). It remains to be proven that such excitation can occur beneath the threshold for activation of nociceptive afferents. Furthermore, the discharge of many slowly conducting, *non-nociceptive* group III-IV mechanoreceptor afferents has been shown to exhibit a *decline* in their discharge during the initial phase of fatigue (Hayward et al. 1991).

At this stage, there is clearly need for a multi-laboratory attack on this issue using both experimental paradigms. For work on conscious humans that test for involvement of group III-IV afferents in the wisdom phenomenon, it will be a formidable problem to discriminate (with microneurography) unitary activity in group III-IV afferents supplying a fatiguing muscle and prove whether the axons subserve nociceptive *vs.* ergoreceptive (exercise related) function (Hasan & Stuart 1984). In the case of reduced-animal experimentation, there are also formidable technical difficulties when recording the activity of single group III-IV afferents (particularly those signaling non-noxious events); but nevertheless, a substantial data base was recently assembled on a somewhat analogous problem (afferent discharge from control vs. inflamed joints; Grigg et al. 1986). Hence, the prospects are promising that a more complete understanding is attainable of the responses of group III-IV chemoreceptor and mechanoreceptor afferents in fatiguing muscle before and after the onset of pain.

Such group III-IV involvement must also be considered in relation to the potential contribution from large diameter group I-II mechanoreceptor afferents. For example, because motor units in humans do not exhibit a decline in discharge rate during sustained activity (brought on by several means) until recovery from anesthetic block is complete, Bongiovanni and Hagbarth (1990) proposed that the decline in discharge rate from a high value is a result of disfacilitation (i.e., reduced post-synaptic excitation of motoneurones via a reduction in fusimotor-driven feedback from muscle spindles; cf. also Gandevia et al. 1990; Macefield et al 1992). This possibility has been supported by evidence showing a fatigue-induced decline in the firing rate of human muscle spindle afferents (Macefield et al. 1991), but the relative roles of reflex inhibition mediated by small diameter afferents and disfacilitation of motoneurones is unresolved. As work continues on this problem, the temporal aspects of muscle wisdom will require special consideration. For example, there is need to evaluate the recent suggestion that *"...One plausible way to amalgamate the current findings is to suggest that any decline in motoneurone discharge rate during the first 5-10s of a maximal voluntary contraction may reflect the reduction in muscle spindle input and increase in presynaptic inhibition, while metabolic effects exerted reflexly through small-diameter afferents contribute more later in the contraction" (Gandevia 1990).*

At present, there is a limited and conflicting set of observations on the effects of fatigue on the sensitivity of large diameter, mechanoreceptor afferents and their spinal-reflex efficacy. For muscle spindle afferent (Ia and spII) sensitivity, the initial results on reduced animals are generally in agreement, with fatigue shown to enhance their responsiveness to single motor unit contractions (Christakos & Windhorst 1986; Enoka et al. 1990; cf. also the 1985 work of Nelson & Hutton on spindle responses to whole muscle stretch). However, of similar merit is evidence from experiments on humans that fatigue results in a decline of fusimotor drive to muscle spindles and consequently reduces spindle discharge (vide supra). For tendon organ (Ib) afferents, the effects of fatigue are also uncertain. In studies on reduced animals, there is evidence of little (Stephens et al. 1975) or no (Gregory 1990) change in their responsiveness to single motor unit contractions; whereas, in similar preparations, there is equally convincing evidence of a reduction in Ib responsiveness to whole muscle stretch (Hutton & Nelson 1986). Similar uncertainty abounds concerning the spinal-reflex efficacy of this sensory input. On the one hand, there is evidence that fatigue enhances the efficacy of short and long latency reflex EMG and motoneurone responses to brief muscle perturbations in humans (Darling & Hayes 1983; Kirsch & Rymer 1987) and reduced animals (Windhorst et al. 1986). However, these results are in possible conflict with those reported for humans by Hunter and Kearney (1983), Crago and Zacharkiw (1985) and Balestra et al. (1992). As this field of investigation continues, studies will be required on the effects of contraction of type-identified motor units on afferent fibers during fatigue in both reduced animals (i.e., as introduced by Stephens et al. 1975) and conscious humans. In the latter instance, a valuable stimulation technique (Westling et al. 1990) has already been applied to the study of motor unit fatigue (Thomas et al. 1991). Also, our understanding of the effects of fatigue on spinal reflex transmission requires analysis of interneuronal pathways (cf. interneuronal wisdom; vide supra) in the conscious human, making use of refined conditioning volley/test shock techniques (e.g., Fournier & Pierrot-Deseilligny 1989) that derive their inspiration from the virtuosic work of the Lundberg group (Baldissera et al. 1981; Jankowska 1992).

On the basis of our current understanding of the spinal actions of muscle afferents, we would propose that any *precise* matching of motoneurone discharge to the stimulus frequency-force relation of its fatiguing muscle unit, on a moment-to-moment basis, is more likely to be attributable to the action of large diameter spindle afferents rather than small diameter ones, with the latter's input providing a more general, sustained inhibition (firing rate reduction) of motoneurone discharge. This speculation is summarized in Fig. 1. It is based on our interpretation of evidence generated largely by Lundberg and Jankowska and their colleagues on the spinal connectivity patterns of limb afferents in reduced cat preparations (reviewed in: Baldissera et al. 1981; McCrea 1996; Stuart 1986; Schomburg 1990; Jankowska 1992).

In considering the implications for the sensory-feedback hypothesis of the organizational scheme proposed in Fig. 1, it must be recognized, of course, that far more is known about the spinal connectivity patterns of group III-IV afferents in cutaneous than in muscle nerves. However, there is evidence that under selected circumstances, such cutaneous input can combine with large diameter, muscle afferent input to achieve a relatively private (concentrated) effect on a particular population of motoneurones (for review: McCrea 1992; Jankowska 1992; cf. also He et al. 1988; Ferrell et al. 1988). Hence, the possibility can not be dismissed at this time, that under the conditions that bring on muscle fatigue, some specialized effects from homonymous, non-nociceptive group III-IV afferent input can be exerted on motoneurones which drive the fatiguing muscle. However, it is parsimonious to consider that this possibility is far less likely than our proposition that a precise reflex control of motoneurone firing rate is far more likely to be attributable to changes in Ia afferent input, with a tonic inhibition progressively building as brought on by the non-nociceptive group III-IV input. Once pain sets in, it is also unlikely that the nociceptor input exerts a private-line effect on homonymous motoneurones or that it could regulate their firing rate in attune with the changing mechanical status of the fatiguing muscle.

As a final reflection on the sensory-feedback hypothesis, it is important to remember that fatigue occurs during sustained and intermittent activation of muscle; it is part and parcel of the numerous problems that must be solved by the CNS in its overall control of movement. The viewpoint has been advanced by Lundberg and Jankowska and their colleagues that *no* one *single* afferent species dominates in the effect of afferent feedback on movement. Rather, the evidence to date points to the scheme we have outlined in Fig. 1: the role of peripheral afferent input from active muscles during fatigue is to support descending command signals that are mediated largely by interneurons on which the majority of afferent input converges. Their argument that *"...it seems much more sensible that different receptors which can give useful information combine in the feedback control and this is best achieved by convergence on interneurons in a common reflex pathway"* (Jankowska & Lundberg 1981) should well apply to fatigue with the added proviso that as fatigue ensues, the reflex control will be influenced to a progressively greater extent by group III-IV sensory input that, itself, becomes progressively more dominated by the nociceptive input.

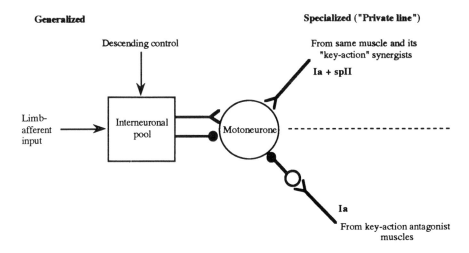

Figure 1. *Overall organization of the central connections and actions of limb afferents.* Shown is a generalized hindlimb extensor motoneurone receiving excitation (—<) and inhibition (—•) from a generalized interneuronal pool responsive to descending control and afferent input from the *entire* limb. In addition, the motoneurones of each single muscle receive relatively discrete (specialized, private line) monosynaptic Ia and spII excitation from their own muscle and its close synergists, and somewhat less discrete disynaptic inhibition (the open circle is generalized in this pathway). These pathways, too, are subject to controls emanating from the generalized interneuronal pool. In this schema, note that the Ia input projects both directly (as shown) to the motoneurone and indirectly (not shown) via the limb afferent input. Also, the interneurons providing disynaptic inhibition to the motoneurone are, in reality, a part of the generalized interneuronal pool.

The Fig. 1 model is based on four lines of evidence:
1. By far the majority of limb afferent input to the spinal cord (including that from Ia and spII afferents) is directed to spinal interneurons on which the descending command signals also converge. The output of this massive interneuronal pool effects motor pools (nuclei) supplying the whole limb. This convergent-divergent arrangement of interneuronal connectivity suggests that sensory input from single muscles contribute more to the integrated control of the limb rather than the singular control of their same (homonymous) muscle.
2. While the mechanical status of single muscles is signaled accurately by the combined ensemble input from their spindles (Ia, spII) and tendon organs (Ib), the central actions of the Ib and shared Ia-Ib feedback (the latter onto interneurons receiving monosynaptic excitation from both Ia and Ib afferents) suggest that their role is to ensure the integrated

actions of many muscles across several joints, rather than to the exclusive regulation of a single muscle.

3. The possibility of an exclusive ("private line"; cf. McCrea 1992) mechanoreceptor reflex control of the homonymous muscle (or, at least, of it and its close synergists) is limited to that derived from the monosynaptic input of Ia and spII afferents. This arrangement is present in most but not all muscle systems, and it, too, is subject, under certain conditions, to a presynaptic inhibitory control from the interneuronal pool (see Rudomin's chapter in Binder & Mendell 1990).

4. A degree of exclusivity may also be provided in disynaptic reciprocal inhibitory pathways activated by Ia afferent input. While interneuronal modulation is ever-present in this pathway, the spinal connectivity pattern of this pathway is at least suggestive of some focus of attention (specialization) on a selected group of muscles, rather than that of the entire limb.

Proprioceptive usage in motor control in the presence of muscle fatigue

As a final comment, we would propose that while the systematic testing of the sensory-feedback hypothesis will contribute to our understanding of segmental motor mechanisms, the study of muscle fatigue has even broader implications for the control of movement. For example, experimental evidence derived from several invertebrate and vertebrate species, performing a wide variety of tasks, now suggests several roles for proprioceptive information (Hasan & Stuart 1988). Table 1 summarizes these roles which are exhibited during sensorimotor integration at *all* levels of the CNS, including the operation of segmental reflexes (***Note:*** Proprioceptors are the receptors that respond to the mechanical variable associated with muscles and joints. In the strictest sense, the proprioceptors have an adequate stimulus that arises from the actions of the organism itself and they include muscle spindles, Golgi tendon organs, and joint receptors in vertebrates, and a variety of stretch receptors and chordotonal organs in invertebrates. In contrast, exteroceptors such as tactile receptors respond primarily to external stimuli. However, the force-sensitive receptors in the exoskeleton of many invertebrates can function as proprioceptors).

An intriguing feature of Table 1 is that neurophysiologists have focused almost exclusively on **only two** of the proposed roles (1.1 & 2.1 in Table 1), with the sensory-feedback hypothesis fitting most closely with studies of conventional reflex testing (i.e., 2.1 in Table 1; appropriate responses to unexpected perturbations). It will be of great utility and interest to arrive at a more complete understanding of the effects of muscle fatigue on the functions summarized in Table 1, and on many other motor functions, as well, when the non-proprioceptive group III-IV input and suprasegmental aspects of muscle fatigue are also taken into account.

Table 1. The role of proprioceptors in motor control

1. Three roles arise from mechanics of the musculoskeletal system. They involve *smoothing* and *stabilizing* of *internally generated* programs.

    1.1 linearization of (correction for) muscle properties

    1.2 compensation for lever-arm variations

    1.3 correction of interjoint interaction effects

2. Three additional roles arise from *interactions* between the *mechanics* of the musculoskeletal system and the *physical environment*.

    2.1 appropriate responses to unexpected perturbations

    2.2 selections of appropriate synergies of response

    2.3 assist external forces, particularly in interlimb coordination

Summary

Muscle wisdom and its proposed sensory-feedback mechanism provide a new opening in the study of muscle fatigue and the function of the segmental motor system, particularly in regard to the neuromuscular control of glycolytic, rapidly fatiguing muscle cells. Numerous experiments on both reduced animal preparations in a wide variety of species and conscious humans are necessary on: *motoneurones,* the relationship between their adaptive properties, size principle issues and mechanisms of motor unit fatigue; *motor units,* associations between the magnitude of fatigue-induced slowing in force-relaxation rate and motoneurone firing rate, recruitment order, force and fatigability; *muscle receptors,* effects of fatigue on their adaptive and transducing properties and; *spinal reflexes,* fatigue-induced modulation of reflex efficacy. In addition, the broad and multifaceted role of proprioceptive usage in the control of movement (also, in a wide variety of species) should now be examined in the presence of muscle fatigue. Clearly, an increased emphasis on the study of muscle fatigue, as guided by clearly defined and perceived issues, will contribute greatly to further advances in our understanding of the segmental motor system, particularly if the work is also stimulated by the spirit of adventurous speculation advanced in this article!

Acknowledgments: The authors wish to thank Drs. Edmund Arbas and Ziaul Hasan for reviewing the manuscript, and Ms. Pat Pierce for her help with manuscript preparation. Our recent work on muscle fatigue has been undertaken in collaboration with Drs. Bevan, Laouris, Enoka, Nemeth, Nordstrom, Robinson and Spielmann, and Mr. Reinking. All their efforts are gratefully appreciated. Our work on fatigue is supported by U.S.P.H.S grants NS 25077 (to D.G.Stuart), NS 20544 (to R.M. Enoka), NS 20762 (to P. Nemeth and R.M. Enoka), HL 07249 (to the Dept. of Physiology), NS 07309 (Motor Control Training Program) and GM 08400 (Physiological Sciences Training Program).

References

Baldissera F, Hultborn H & Illert M (1981). Integration in spinal neuronal systems. In: *Handbook of Physiology, sec. 1, vol. II, pt. 1. The Nervous System: Motor Control.* Brooks VB (vol. ed.) Eds, Brookhart JM & Mountcastle VB. American Physiological Society. Bethesda. pp 509-595.

Balestra C, Dachateau J & Hainaut (1992). Effects of fatigue on the stretch reflex in a human muscle. *Electroencephalography & Clinical Neurophysiology* In press.

Bergstrom M & Hultman E (1988). Energy cost and fatigue during intermittent electrical stimulation of human skeletal muscle. *Journal of Applied Physiology* **65,** 1500-1505.

Bevan L, Laouris Y, Reinking RM & Stuart DG (1992). The effect of the stimulation pattern on the fatigue of single motor units in adult cats. *Journal of Physiology* **449,** 85-108.

Bigland-Ritchie BR, Dawson NJ, Johansson RS & Lippold OCJ (1986). Reflex origin for the slowing of motoneurone firing rates in fatigue of human voluntary contractions. *Journal of Physiology* **379,** 451-459.

Bigland-Ritchie BR, Johansson R, Lippold OCJ, Smith S & Woods JJ (1983). Changes in motoneurone firing rates during sustained maximal voluntary contractions. *Journal of Physiology* **340,** 335-346.

Binder MD & Mendell LM (1990). *The Segmental Motor System.* Oxford University Press. New York.

Binder-Macleod SA & Barker CB III (1991). Use of a catch-like property of human skeletal muscle to reduce fatigue. *Muscle & Nerve* **14,** 850-857.

Binder-Macleod SA & McDermond LR (1992). Changes in the force-frequency relationship of the human quadriceps muscle following electrically and voluntarily induced fatigue. *Physical Therapy* **72,** 95-104.

Bongiovanni LG & Hagbarth K-H (1990). Tonic vibration reflexes elicited during fatigue from maximum voluntary contractions in man. *Journal of Physiology* **423,** 1-15.

Botterman BR & Cope TC (1988). Maximum tension predicts relative endurance of fast-twitch motor units in the cat. *Journal of Neurophysiology* **60,** 1215-1226.

Brownstone RM, Jordan, Kriellaars DJ, Noga BR & Shefchyk SJ (1992). On the regulation of repetitive firing in lumbar motoneurones during fictive locomotion in the cat. *Experimental Brain Research* In press.

Callister RJ, Reinking RM & Stuart DG (1992). The effect of fatigue on the catch-like property of turtle skeletal muscle. *Western Nerve Net Meeting, San Diego, CA, March 27-29*.

Christakos CN & Windhorst U (1986). Spindle gain increase during muscle unit fatigue. *Brain Research* **365**, 388-392.

Cooper RG, Edwards RHT, Gibson H & Stokes MJ (1988). Human muscle fatigue: frequency dependence of excitation and force generation. *Journal of Physiology* **397**, 585-599.

Crago PE & Zacharkiw SV (1985). Lack of stretch reflex compensation for fatigue induced changes in stiffness of the flexor pollicus longus. *Society for Neuroscience Abstracts* **11**, 213.

Czeh G, Gallego R, Kudo N & Kuno M (1978). Evidence for the maintenance of motoneurone properties by muscle activity. *Journal of Physiology* **281**, 239-252.

Darling WG & Hayes KC (1983). Human servo responses to load disturbances in fatigued muscle. *Brain Research* **267**, 345-351.

Dietz V (1978). Analysis of the electrical muscle activity during maximal contraction and the influence of ischaemia. *Journal of Neurological Sciences* **37**, 187-197.

Dubose L, Schelhorn TB & Clamann HP (1987). Changes in contractile speed of cat motor units during activity. *Muscle & Nerve* **10**, 744-752.

Duchateau J & Hainaut K (1985). Electrical and mechanical failure during sustained and intermittent contractions in humans. *Journal of Applied Physiology* **58**, 942-947.

Edwards RHT (1981). Human muscle function and fatigue. In: *Human Muscle Fatigue: Physiological Mechanisms* Eds, Porter R & Whelan J. Pitman Medical. London. pp 1-18.

Enoka RM, Nordstrom MA, Reinking RM & Stuart DG (1990). Motor unit-muscle spindle interactions during fatigue. *Society for Neuroscience Abstracts* **16**, 886.

Enoka RM & Stuart DG (1992). Neurobiology of muscle fatigue. *Journal of Applied Physiology* In press.

Ferrell WR, Wood L & Baxendale RH (1988). The effect of acute joint inflammation on flexion reflex excitability in the decerebrate low-spinal cat. *Quarterly Journal of Physiology* **73**, 95-102.

Fournier E & Pierrot-Deseilligny P (1989). Changes in transmission in some reflex pathways during movement in humans. *News in Physiological Sciences* **4**, 29-32.

Gandevia SC (1990). Neuromuscular fatigue mechanisms: central and peripheral factors affecting motoneuronal output in fatigue. In: *Fatigue in Sports and Exercise* F.I.T. Victoria University of Technology. Footscray, Australia. pp 9-15.

Gandevia SC, Macefield G, Burke D & McKenzie DK (1990). Voluntary activation of human motor axons in the absence of muscle afferent feedback. The control of the deafferented hand. *Brain* **113**, 1563-1581.

Gardiner PF & Kernell LD (1990). The "fastness" of rat motoneurones: time-course of afterhyperpolarization in relation to axonal conduction velocity and muscle unit contractile speed. *Pflügers Archiv. European Journal of Physiology* **415**, 762-766.

Garland SJ (1991). Role of small diameter afferents in reflex inhibition during human muscle fatigue. *Journal of Physiology* **435**, 547-558.

Garland SJ, Garner SH & McComas AJ (1988). Reduced voluntary electromyographic activity after fatiguing stimulation of human muscle. *Journal of Physiology* **401**, 547-556.

Garland SJ & McComas AJ (1990). Reflex inhibition of human soleus muscle during fatigue. *Journal of Physiology* **429**, 17-27.

Gielen CCAM, Ramaekers L & van Zuylen EJ (1988). Long-latency stretch reflexes as co-ordinated functional responses in man. *Journal of Physiology* **407**, 275-292.

Giszter SF, McIntyre J & Bizzi E (1989). Kinematic strategies and sensorimotor transformations in the wiping movements of frogs. *Journal of Neurophysiology* **62**, 750-767.

Gordon DA, Enoka RM, Karst GM & Stuart DG (1990). Force development and relaxation in single motor units of adult cats during a standard fatigue test. *Journal of Physiology* **421**, 583-594.

Gregory JE (1990). Relations between identified tendon organs and motor units in the medial gastrocnemius muscle of the cat. *Experimental Brain Research* **81**, 602-608.

Grigg P, Schaible HG & Schmidt RF (1986). Mechanical sensitivity of group III-IV afferents from posterior articular nerve in normal and inflamed knee. *Journal of Neurophysiology* **55,** 635-643.

Grillner S, Buchanan JT, Wallén P & Brodin L (1988). Neural control of locomotion in lower vertebrates. In: *Neural Control of Rhythmic Movements in Vertebrates*. Eds, Cohen A, Rossignol S & Grillner S. John Wiley & Sons, Inc. New York. pp 1-40.

Grillner S, Wallén P, Brodin L & Lansner A (1991). Neural network generating locomotor behavior in lamprey: circuitry, transmitters, membrane properties, and simulation. *Annual Review of Neuroscience* **14,** 169-199.

Gurfinkel VS, Levik YS, Popov KE, Smetanin BN & Shlikov VY (1988). Body scheme in the control of postural activity. In: *Stance and Motion, Facts and Concepts*. Eds, Gurfinkel VS, Ioffe ME, Massion J & Roll JP. Plenum Press. New York. pp 185-193.

Hasan Z & Stuart DG (1984). Mammalian Muscle Receptors. In: *Handbook of the Spinal Cord, Vols. 2 and 3, Anatomy and Physiology*. Ed, Davidoff RA. Marcel Dekker. New York. pp 559-607.

Hasan Z & Stuart DG (1988). Animal solutions to problems of movement control: the role of proprioceptors. *Annual Review of Neuroscience* **11,** 199-223.

Hayward L, Wesselmann U & Rymer WZ (1991). Effects of muscle fatigue on mechanically sensitive afferents of slow conduction velocity in the cat triceps surae. *Journal of Neurophysiology* **65,** 360-370.

He X, Proske U, Schaible H-G, Schmidt, RF (1988). Acute inflammation of the knee joint in the cat alters responses of flexor motoneurones to leg movements. *Journal of Neurophysiology* **59,** 326-340.

Hounsgaard J, Kiehn O & Mintz I (1988). Response properties of motoneurones in a slice preparation of the turtle spinal cord. *Journal of Physiology* **398,** 575-589.

Hunter IW & Kearney RE (1983). Invariance of ankle dynamic stiffness during fatiguing muscle contractions. *Journal of Biomechanics* **16,** 985-991.

Hutton RS & Nelson DL (1986). Stretch sensitivity of Golgi tendon organs in fatigued gastrocnemius muscle. *Medicine and Science in Sports and Exercise* **18,** 69-74.

Jankowska, E (1992). Interneuronal relay in spinal pathways from proprioceptors. *Progress in Neurobiology* **38,** 335-378.

Jankowska E & Lundberg A (1981). Interneurons in the spinal cord. *Trends in Neurosciences* **4,** 230-233.

Kaufmann MP, Rotto DM & Rybicki KJ (1988). Pressor reflex responses to static muscular contraction: its afferent arm and possible neurotransmitters. *American Journal of Cardiology* **62,** 58E-62E.

Kernell D & Monster AW (1982a). Time course and properties of late adaptation in spinal motoneurones of the cat. *Experimental Brain Research* **46,** 191-196.

Kernell D & Monster AW (1982b). Motoneurone properties and motor fatigue: An intracellular study of gastrocnemius motoneurones of the cat. *Experimental Brain Research* **46,** 197-204.

Kirsch RF & Rymer WZ (1987). Neural compensation for muscular fatigue: evidence for significant force regulation in man. *Journal of Neurophysiology* **57,** 1893-1910.

Kniffki K-D, Mense S & Schmidt RF (1981). Muscle receptors with fine afferent fibers which may evoke circulatory reflexes. *Circulation Research* **48,** 125-131.

Koshland GF, Gerilovsky L & Hasan Z (1991). Activity of wrist muscles during imposed or voluntary movements about the elbow joint. *Journal of Motor Behavior* **23,** 91-100.

Kukulka CG, Russell AG & Moore MA (1986). Electrical and mechanical changes in human soleus muscle during sustained maximum isometric contractions. *Brain Research* **362,** 47-54.

Lacquaniti F, Borghese NA & Carrozzo M (1991). Transient reversal of stretch reflex in human muscles. *Journal of Neurophysiology* **66,** 939-954.

Llinas R & Lopez-Barneo J (1988). Electrophysiology of mammalian tectal neurons in vitro. II. Long-term adaptation. *Journal of Neurophysiology* **60,** 869-878.

Macefield G, Gandevia SC, Bigland-Ritchie B, Groman R & Burke D (1992). The discharge rate of human motoneurones innervating ankle dorsiflexors in the absence of muscle afferent feedback. *Journal of Physiology* In press.

Macefield G, Hagbarth K-E, Gorman R, Gandevia SC & Burke D (1991). Decline in spindle support to α-motoneurones during sustained voluntary contractions. *Journal of Physiology* **440,** 497-512.

Marsden CD, Meadows JD & Merton PA (1976). Fatigue in human muscle in relation to the number and frequency of motor impulses. *Journal of Physiology* **258,** 94P.

Marsden CD, Meadows JC & Merton PA (1983). "Muscular wisdom" that minimizes fatigue during prolonged effort in man: Peak rates of motoneuron discharge and slowing of discharge during fatigue. In: *Motor Control Mechanisms in Health and Disease.* Ed, Desmedt, JE. Raven Press. New York. pp 169-211.

McCrea DA (1992). Can sense be made of spinal interneuron circuits? *Behavioral Brain Science* In press.

McKenzie DK & Gandevia SC (1991). Recovery from fatigue of human diaphragm and limb muscles. *Respiratory Physiology* **84,** 49-60.

Nelson DL & Hutton RS (1985). Dynamic and static stretch responses in muscle spindle receptors in fatigued muscle. *Medicine and Science in Sports and Exercise* **17,** 445-450.

Nordstrom MA, Spielmann JM, Laouris Y, Reinking RM & Stuart DG (1991). Motor-neuron adaptation in response to intermittent extracellular activation. *Abstracts, Third IBRO World Congress of Neuroscience, Montréal, Canada, August 4-7* 407.

Ogata T (1988). Morphological and cytochemical features of fiber types in vertebrate skeletal muscle. *CRC Critical Reviews in Anatomy and Cell Biology* **1,** 229-275.

Ostry DJ, Feldman AG & Flanagan JR (1991). Kinematics and control of frog hindlimb movements. *Journal of Neurophysiology* **65,** 547-562.

Rathmayer W & Maier L (1987). Muscle fiber types in crabs: studies on single identified muscle fibers. *American Zoology* **27,** 1067-1077.

Rome LC, Funke RP, Alexander RM, Lutz G, Aldridge H, Scott F & Freadman M (1988). Why animals have different muscle fibre types. *Nature* **335,** 824-827.

Rotto DM & Kaufmann MP (1988). Effect of metabolic products of muscular contraction on discharge of group III and IV afferents. *Journal of Applied Physiology* **64,** 2306-2313.

Schomburg ED (1990). Spinal sensorimotor systems and their supraspinal control *Neuroscience Research* **7,** 265-340.

Spielmann JM (1991). *Quantification of motor-neuron adaptation to sustained and intermittent stimulation. (Ph.D. thesis, Univ. Microfilm Int. Cit. No. 9123464).* University of Arizona. Tucson, AZ, USA.

Spielmann JM, Laouris Y, Nordstrom MA, Reinking RM & Stuart DG (1990). Time course of motoneuronal adaptation in response to extracellular activation with superimposed pink noise. *Society for Neuroscience Abstracts* **16,** 114.

Spielmann JM, Nordstrom MA, Laouris Y & Stuart DG (1991). The relation between motor-neuron adaptation and muscle fatigue. *Abstracts, Third IBRO World Congress of Neuroscience, Montréal, Canada, August 4-7* 407.

Stephens JA, Reinking RM & Stuart DG (1975). The tendon organs of cat medial gastrocnemius: Responses to active and passive forces as a function of muscle length. *Journal of Physiology* **38,** 1217-1231.

Stuart DG (1985). Summary and challenges for future work. In: *Motor Control: From Movement Trajectories to Neural Mechanisms. Short Course Syllabus.* Society for Neuroscience. Bethesda, MD. pp 95-105.

Stuart DG (1986). Mammalian muscle receptors. In: *Loaded Breathing: Load Compensation and Respiratory Sensation.* (F.A.S.E.B. Symposium Summary) Eds, Altose MD, Zechman FW Jr. *Fed. Proc.* pp 114-122.

Stuart DG & Enoka RM (1983). Motoneurons, motor units, and the size principle. In: *The Clinical Neurosciences, Sec. 5, Neurobiology. (Willis WD, Sec. ed.)* Ed, Rosenberg RN. Churchill Livingstone. New York. pp 471-517.

Stuart DG & Enoka RM (1990). Henneman's contributions in historical perspective. In: *Segmental Motor System.* Eds, Binder MD & Mendell LM. Oxford University Press. New York. pp 3-19.

Thomas CK, Johansson RS & Bigland-Ritchie B (1991). Attempts to physiologically classify human thenar motor units. *Journal of Neurophysiology* **65,** 1501-1508.

Vrbová G (1989). The concept of neuromuscular plasticity. *Journal of Neurology and Rehabilitation* **3,** 1-6.

Westling G, Johansson RS, Thomas CK & Bigland-Ritchie B (1990). Measurement of contractile and electrical properties of single human thenar motor units in response to intraneural motor-axon stimulation. *Journal of Neurophysiology* **64,** 1331-1337.

Windhorst U, Christakos CN, Koehler W, Hamm TM, Enoka RM & Stuart DG (1986). Amplitude reduction of motor unit twitches during repetitive activation is accompanied by relative increase of hyperpolarizing membrane potential trajectories in homonymous α-motoneurons. *Brain Research* **398,** 181-184.

Woods JJ, Furbush F & Bigland-Ritchie B (1987). Evidence for a fatigue induced reflex inhibition of motoneuron firing rates. *Journal of Neurophysiology* **58,** 125-137.

Zhang L & Krnjevic K (1987). Apamin depresses selectively the after-hyperpolarization of cat spinal motoneurons. *Neuroscience Letters* **74,** 58-62.

Multiple neuromuscular-strategies for counteracting muscle fatigue

Yiannis Laouris*+ & Douglas G. Stuart*

+Department of Neural Control, Cyprus Neuroscience & Technology Institute,
Lycourgou 10/401, Acropolis, Nicosia Cyprus.
*Department of Physiology, College of Medicine, University of Arizona, Tucson,
Arizona 85724 USA.

In recent years, there has been much interest in the possibility that a slowing of whole-muscle contractile speed (particularly force relaxation), which lowers fusion frequency, is matched by a slowing of motoneuronal discharge to result in an enhancement ("optimization") of force production (Bigland-Ritchie et al. 1983; Dietz et al. 1978; Marsden et al. 1983), particularly in glycolytic rapidly fatiguing components of the muscle (cf. Stuart & Callister, this volume), and a delay in the onset of central fatigue (Enoka & Stuart 1992), at least in the short range. In this report, we focus on two additional strategies available to the neuromuscular system to reduce and delay fatigue, also on at least a short-range basis: increased non-linearities in temporal force summation, and increased variability of motoneuronal discharge.

Increase of nonlinearities in temporal force summation

Our group has recently compared the force responses of glycolytic, rapidly fatiguing motor units of the adult cat to repetitive (1/s) stimulation with a regular pattern (interpulse interval = 1.8 times contraction time; duration 400 or 500 ms) vs. an "optimized" pattern (same number of stimuli delivered over same time, but rearranged to optimize force in the pre-fatigue state), using pseudo-random alternation of the two patterns (Bevan et al. 1992; Laouris et al. 1989). The results showed that the optimized pattern not only produced more force at all times throughout the test, but the relative amount of force enhancement increased (up to 200%) as fatigue ensued. This result, involving an interaction between fatigue and the catch-like property of mammalian muscle cells, can be considered an example of the use of an increase in non-linear force summation to reduce and delay fatigue. A more recent experiment in our laboratory has revealed that the turtle muscle also exhibits the catch-like property, and that it, too, is enhanced following fatiguing stimulation (Callister et al. 1992). We consider this finding particularly intriguing, because it suggests that the neuromuscular strategy of increasing non-linear force summation may have been subject to evolutionary conservation (Stuart & Callister, this volume) as a means of reducing and delaying fatigue in life-threatening situations.

Increase of motoneuron discharge variability

In addition to a fatigue-induced decline in motor unit activation rates, several studies on humans have suggested that these rates also exhibit an increase of their variability of interpulse interval (Gatev et al. 1986; Enoka et al. 1989; Nordstrom & Miles, 1990). In a reduced-animal preparation, our group has recently shown that following two minutes of constant-current extracellular stimulation, the normalized discharge variability of spinal motoneurones of the adult cat increased linearly with time (in preparation; see also Laouris et al. 1990). This increase is attributed to intrinsic (biophysical) properties of the motoneuron, rather than extrinsic (synaptically mediated) ones, because the animals were under deep pentobarbital anaesthesia and the spinal dorsal roots were cut. Our ongoing analysis is testing:

1) whether this fatigue-induced intrinsic increase in discharge variability may be augmented by an increase in synaptic noise; 2) for associations with size-related properties of the motor unit, including the same motoneurones' firing rate adaptations to sustained (Spielmann et al. 1990) and intermittent (Nordstrom et al. 1991) stimulation, and the fatigability of their motor units.

Summary and Conclusions

Although first observed at least fifty years ago (Seyffarth 1940), there is only recent interest in observations that the behaviour (strategy) of the neuromuscular system changes during fatiguing muscle contractions in a manner that tends to reduce and delay fatigue, particularly of the rapidly fatiguing glycolytic, muscle cells. The strategies considered to this point, matched rates of motoneurone firing and motor unit force relaxation, increased nonlinearity in temporal force summation, and increased variability of motoneurone discharge are probably not the only ones available to the CNS and the peripheral neuromuscular system. However, the study of the mechanisms underlying these strategies and their interrelationships, should stimulate enhanced interest in how the CNS solves its motor-control problems in both the fresh and fatigued state.

Acknowledgements

Our recent work on temporal force summation and motoneurone firing properties has been undertaken in collaboration with Drs. Bevan, Callister, Nordstrom, Robinson and Spielmann, and Mr. Reinking. All their efforts are gratefully appreciated. Our work on fatigue is supported by USPHS grants NS 25077 (to DGS), NS 20544 (to R.M. Enoka), NS 20762 (to P. Nemeth and R.M. Enoka), HL 07249 (to the Dept. of Physiology), NS 07309 (Motor Control Training Program) and GM 08400 (Physiological Sciences Training Program).

References

Bevan, L, Laouris, Y, Reinking, R. & Stuart, DG (1992). The effect of the stimulation pattern on the fatigue of single motor units in adult cats. *Journal of Physiology* (in press).

Bigland-Ritchie, B, Johansson, R, Lippold, OC, Smith, S & Woods, JJ (1983). Changes in motoneurone firing rates during sustained maximal voluntary contractions. *Journal of Physiology* **340**, 335-346.

Callister, RJ, Reinking, R. & Stuart, DG (1992). The effect of fatigue on the catch-like property of turtle muscle. Western Nerve Net Meeting, San Diego, California, Mar. 27-29.

Dietz, V (1978). Analysis of the electrical muscle activity during maximal contraction and the influence of ischaemia. *Journal of Neurological Sciences* **37**, 187-197.

Enoka, RM, Robinson, GA & Kossev, AR (1989). Task and fatigue effects on low-threshold motor units in human hand muscle. *Journal of Neurophysiology* **62**, 1344-1359.

Enoka, RM & Stuart, DG (1992). Neurobiology of muscle fatigue. *Journal of Applied Physiology* (in press).

Gatev, P, Ivanova, T. & Gantchev, GN (1986). Changes in the firing pattern of high-threshold motor units due to fatigue. *Electromyography and Clinical Neurophysiology* **26**, 83-93.

Laouris, Y, Bevan, L, Reinking, RM & Stuart, DG. (1989). The force:fatigability relationship in single motor units: 2. A new experimental paradigm supported by simulations. *Abstracts Society of Neuroscience* **15**, 396.

Laouris, Y, Bevan, L, Spielmann, JM, Nordstrom, MA, Reinking, RM & Stuart, DG. (1990). Changes in motoneuron discharge variability during prolonged activation with extracellular stimulation: possible implications for fatigue. In: *Muscle Fatigue Biochemical and Physiological Aspects*, ed. Atlan, G, Belivea, L &Bouissou, P. Paris: Masson, pp. 242.

Marsden, CD, Meadows, JC & Merton, PA (1983). "Muscular wisdom" that minimized fatigue during prolonged effort in man: peak rates of motoneuron discharge and slowing discharge during fatigue. In: *Motor Control Mechanisms in Health and Disease*, ed. Desmedt, J.E. Raven. New York. pp 169-211.

Nordstrom & Miles (1990). Fatigue of single motor units in human masseter. *Journal of Applied Physiology* **68**, 26-34.

Nordstrom, MA, Spielmann, JM, Laouris, Y, Reinking, RM & Stuart, DG (1991). Motor neuron adaptation in response to intermittent extracellular activation. *Abstracts, Third IBRO World Congress of Neuroscience* (Montréal, Canada), p. 111.

Seyffarth, H (1940). The behaviour of motor units in voluntary contractions. *Avhandlinger utgitt av det norske videnskap-akademii Oslo. I. Matematisk-Naturvidenskapelig Klasse* **4**, 1-63.

Spielmann, JM, Laouris, Y, Nordstrom, MA, Reinking, RM & Stuart, DG (1990). Time course of motoneuronal adaptation in response to extracellular activation with superimposed pink noise. *Abstracts Society of Neuroscience* **16**, 114.

Daily "endurance-demands" in cat's ankle muscles

E.Hensbergen and D.Kernell

Department of Neurophysiology, Academisch Medisch Centrum, University of Amsterdam, Meibergdreef 15, 1105 AZ Amsterdam, The Netherlands

Introduction

It is well known that normal muscles are markedly heterogenous with respect to the fatigue resistance of their motor units. In most known kinds of motor behaviour, units with a high degree of endurance are more easily recruited than those that are more fatigue-sensitive. Hence, the high-endurance units will be more heavily used per day or, in other words, they face a greater daily "endurance-demand" in terms of cumulative daily activity time.

Altered endurance-demands lead to long-term changes in fatigue resistance. Chronic stimulation experiments on cat's pretibial ankle muscles have indicated that endurance becomes markedly improved after a few weeks of extra activity covering 5% of total daily time; 0.5% of such extra duty time was insufficient for increasing endurance (Kernell et al. 1987). This might be taken to suggest that the most heavily used units of a mixed cat muscle would normally be active during at least about 0.5-5% of total daily time.

A greater daily activity time might normally be expected in muscles containing a large percentage of high-endurance units than in those which are relatively more dominated by fatigue-sensitive units. The present experiments were designed for testing these predictions by obtaining activity measurements from muscles that are known from literature to:

1/ contain markedly different percentages of slow-twitch high-endurance units and the corresponding histochemical type of muscle fibre (S-units, type I fibres; percentages are much higher for soleus than for extensor digitorum longus or tibialis anterior; Ariano et al. 1973);

2/ be regionalized in such a way that different muscle portions contain different densities of S-units/type I fibres (in tibialis anterior, such densities are higher for posterior than for anterior portions; Iliya and Dum 1984).

Material & methods

The experimental data were obtained from 4 adult, female cats (weights 2.6-4.1 kg), chronically implanted with bipolar "patch-electrodes" on soleus (anterior side, SOL), extensor digitorum longus (posterior side, EDL), and tibialis anterior (anterior side, TAA; posterior side, TAP). During each recording session of 24 hours, one experimental animal and one cat for company were housed together in a large cage (1x3 m floorspace) within which they could move about freely.

The recordings consisted of telemetrically transmitted electromyographic (EMG) signals from different pairwise combinations of the 4 implanted muscle portions. Each session lasted 24 hr, and the EMG signals from each analyzed muscle pair were then recorded during 48 continuous 4 minute periods, as sampled at half hour intervals. All EMG recordings were saved on tape.

During the subsequent off-line analysis, the EMG signals were rectified and smoothed (time constant 20 ms), and this "integrated EMG" was used to trigger a voltage-level discriminator. For each recording separately, the threshold of the voltage-level discriminator was adjusted to be as low as possible above the baseline noise. The total duration of time that a muscle (portion) were found to be active was expressed in per cent of total recording time, i.e. in a value equivalent to the relative amount of activity per 24 hours for the most active units "seen" by the EMG electrode.

Results and conclusions

1. Cumulative activity times all exceeded 0.5% and were, for most recordings from mixed muscles (TAA, EDL, TAP), in the range 0.5-5% (Fig.1).

2. The cumulative activity times tended to be significantly higher for muscles (muscle portions) known to contain a high percentage of S-units/type-I fibres than for those with smaller fractions of such markedly fatigue-resistant units and fibres (SOL vs. others; TAP vs. TAA; Fig.1).

3. The extreme composition of the cat's soleus muscle (typically 100% slow units and type I fibres) was matched by extreme cumulative activity times of more than twice those seen in the other sampled muscles. The results from soleus resemble those earlier published by Alaimo et al. (1984).

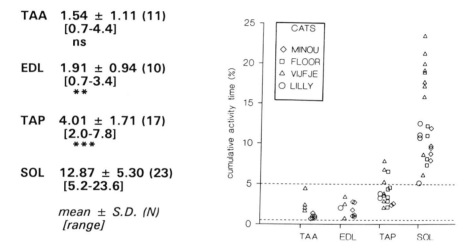

TAA	1.54 ± 1.11 (11)
	[0.7-4.4]
	ns
EDL	1.91 ± 0.94 (10)
	[0.7-3.4]
	**
TAP	4.01 ± 1.71 (17)
	[2.0-7.8]
	***
SOL	12.87 ± 5.30 (23)
	[5.2-23.6]
	mean ± S.D. (N)
	[range]

Figure 1. Numerical (left) and graphical (right) summary of all measured cumulative activity times for four muscle (portions), as expressed in per cent of total recording time. In the numerical section, indications are given of statistical significance of differences between neighbouring rows (t test; ** $P<0.01$, *** $P<0.001$, ns $P>0.4$; for TAA vs. TAP, $P<0.001$). In the graph, different symbols are used for different cats, and interrupted lines are drawn through values of 0.5% and 5%.

References

Alaimo MA, Smith JL, Roy RR & Edgerton VR (1984). EMG activity of slow and fast ankle extensors following spinal cord transection. *Journal of Applied Physiology* **56**, 1608-1613.

Ariano MA, Armstrong RB & Edgerton VR (1973). Hindlimb muscle fiber populations of five mammals. *Journal of Histochemistry and Cytochemistry* **21**, 51-55.

Iliya AR & Dum RP (1984). Somatotopic relations between the motor nucleus and its innervated muscle fibers in the cat tibialis anterior. *Experimental Neurology* **86**, 272-292.

Kernell D, Donselaar Y & Eerbeek O (1987). Effects of physiological amounts of high- and low-rate chronic stimulation on fast-twitch muscle of the cat hindlimb. II. Endurance-related properties. *Journal of Neurophysiology* **58**, 614-627.

Discussions

Discussions

In this section we, the editors, have attempted to summarize the major issues raised during discussions. It is not a verbatim record. We have consolidated some parts of the discussion to avoid repetition, omitted minor points, and omitted purely methodological questions when these are dealt with in the submitted paper. Regrettably, due to technical problems, good quality tape recordings were not available for every session and consequently the report of the discussion of some papers may appear limited - but this does not imply an absence of lively discussion which followed all of the papers.

In producing this summary we thought it sensible to avoid specific attribution of what are editorialised versions of points raised. Nevertheless it should be made clear to the reader that this summary is the outcome of the involvement and enthusiasm of all of the participants and we are indebted to them for taking part and contributing to the success of the symposium.

In planning the meeting we made, we thought, a more than usually generous allowance of time for discussion - but there is never enough time! This was especially the case in relation to the discussion of the supporting papers which were presented as posters. We have not attempted any specific summary of these sessions although many of the major issues raised were common to the discussions summarized below.

CELLULAR PROCESSES OF MUSCLE

In relation to the talk by **Lännergren** it was pointed out:
- that there may still be some uncertainty (particularly for thin mammalian muscle fibres) with respect to the extent to which a sarcolemmal action potential might activate contractile processes directly, without mediation of active propagation of "spikes" along the T tubuli.
- that there is not always a clear association between metabolite levels (e.g. ATP, CP, IMP) and force decline; the force-fatigue may sometimes develop before any marked metabolite changes and, in case of changed metabolite levels, the force may continue to be diminished after normalization of these levels.

In relation to the presentation by **de Haan** and the suggestion that IMP may play a role in fatigue the question was asked what happened in patients with AMP deaminase deficiency? In response it was observed that regulation by IMP would be only one of a number of regulating mechanisms which might act during fatiguing exercise (e.g. changes in Pi and pH). Emphasis was again placed on the fact that *the* process that was limiting in any given situation would be specific to that situation (as determined by: the type of exercise; duty cycle; recruitment pattern; etc.). It was further hypothesised that adaptation may occur due to the absence of any one mechanism so that others become more effective.

The question was raised as to whether *the effects* of glycogen depletion are different between slow and fast fibres. In response it was suggested that although the rates of glycogen degradation are very different between the fibre types the consequences on the energetic status which lead to fatigue might be expected to be the same.

It was also pointed out that an apparent lack of glycogenolysis in type I fibres should be interpreted with care. There was the possibilty that this was the consequence of the chosen stimulation protocol whereby the delay between bouts of stimulation may be sufficient for type I fibres to meet their energy demands via oxidative phosphorylation and PCr resynthesis.

EMG RELATED PROCESSES

In relation to the paper of **McComas** the question was raised as to why fibre hyperpolarization has not been found by previous workers studying muscle fatigue. The explanation may be that most previous workers have not included protein in the solutions bathing their in vitro preparations. It was shown about 30 years ago by Kernan, and by Creese and Northover, that if protein is omitted the sodium permeability of the muscle fibre increases and there is a depolarization of about 10 mV. The general importance of adding protein (and it seems that almost any protein will do the job) to the bathing solution in order to maintain viability of single fibre preparations was underlined.

It was asked whether the slowing of impulse conduction in the muscle fibres secondary to a fall in pH might account for an increase in motor unit potential amplitude. In reponse it was agreed that the effect of impulse slowing could certainly lead to an increase in the *area* of the motor action potential. It seems less certain that it would lead to an increase in peak to peak amplitude: When intracellularly-recorded muscle fibre action potentials start to broaden for any reason there is also a decline in amplitude. Furthermore, since, in the type of experiments described by McComas, ouabain abolishes M wave enlargement, there can be no doubt that the phenomenom is due to electrogenic Na+, K+ pumping.

It was asked whether the effects of interstitial potassium as a stimulant to the sodium potassium pump could be dismissed. Hodgkin and Horowicz were quoted as finding that in their single fibre work adding potassium could sometimes cause a hyperpolarization. In answer it was stated that over most of the range of external potassium concentrations, there is a linear relationship between the logarithm of the latter and the resting membrane potential, more potassium giving less negativity. It might be however that at very low potassium concentrations, where there is some deviation from linearity, the addition of potassium stimulated the pump and restored the electrogenic component of the resting potential.

Finally the question was asked how the noradrenergic fibres would be activated during muscle contractions. It was suggested in response that this might be in one of several ways. It could be by efferent sympathetic drive, associated with motoneuronal activity. Alternatively, it seems possible that the action currents in the extrafusal muscle fibres might passively depolarize the noradrenergic varicosities lying close to them. Finally the rise in interstitial potassium concentration might have a depolarizing effect on the noradrenergic fibres.

In relation to the paper of **De Luca** the question was raised as to how closely the functional, and especially dynamic contractile characteristics, reflected the progressive changes seen in the EMG. This was especially relevant since in many experimental designs rather than a simple progressively developing fatigue, an initial period occurred in which a potentiation of function was seen.

MUSCLE PERFORMANCE - MECHANICAL DEMAND
AND METABOLIC SUPPLY

In relation to the presentation of **Sargeant** an issue which was discussed at some length was the extent to which muscle blood flow may be limiting in fatiguing dynamic exercise. It was pointed out that blood flow could be influenced not only by the duration of the contractions but also by the length of the recovery phase. As a consequence there might be an insufficiency of blood flow both at low and at very high contraction frequencies. An additional point is that as fatigue develops so the time required for relaxation increases, possibly impinging further on the period for unrestricted blood flow.

There was discussion of why the system should continue to recruit slow fibres at very fast pedalling rates when they may make very little contribution to power output and whether there was derecruitment at very high pedalling rates. It might also be thought that a velocity related decline in the efficiency of type I fibres would be an additional reason for recruitment. However the efficiency/velocity and power/velocity relationships of different human fibre types are a matter of extreme speculation, especially as they relate to activities such as running and cycling. In any event there seems to be no evidence *for* derecruitment in these sorts of experiments. Evidence from the pattern of glycogen depletion indicates significant depletion in *all* fibre types in high intensity cycling exercise performed both at 60 and 120 rev/min (see Beelen et al - this volume).

It was also pointed out that the use of standard histochemical techniques to type human muscle fibres may obscure important differences within fibre types, especially when comparing one muscle with another, or the same fibre type in different subjects.

In relation to the presentation of **Jones** the question was raised of the comparability of protocols involving dynamic contractions with repetitive isometric contractions. In response it was pointed out that in brief intermittent contractions of human muscle studied in-situ you cannot make genuinely isometric contractions. The muscle is in fact shortening and the joints moving as substantial work is performed on the elastic and compressive elements of the muscle-tendon-joint complex.

It was asked why the reduction in power in the fatigued muscle should be similar or parallel to the changes in relaxation rate. In was pointed out that relaxation depended on two processes: re-accumulation of calcium; and detachment of cross-bridges. In the fatigued muscle both processes can be affected but slowing in the re-uptake of calcium would not be expected to alter the force-velocity relationship. If, however, the force-velocity relationship does change in fatigue, due to a slowing in the rate of cross bridge detachment, then relaxation rate will also be affected.

It was also pointed out that while calcium transport had been shown to be the rate limiting process for relaxation in resting muscle this was not necessarily the case in the fatigued state.

It was pointed out that the relative magnitude of the fatigue effect on isometric force generation as compared to power production was not constant but depended on the fatiguing protocol. It was commented that it was essential to keep these two aspects of fatigue in mind since you cannot simply deduce one from the other.

The importance of the type and timing of imposed repetitive contractions in relation to the effect of slowed relaxation was raised. The point was made that there was a considerable difference between repeated contractions separated by a clear time interval and those, as often in locomotion, which give little time between contractions for relaxation. Reference was made to the recent work of Curtin and Woledge on fish muscle in which during imposed cyclical contractions the failure to relax fast enough interfered with power production in the following shortening phase.

In relation to the presentation of **Faulkner** there was an extended discussion regarding the comparison of soleus and EDL muscles. Indeed the results of the experiments argued against a prevailing climate of belief that slow muscle (fibres) was much superior to fast in producing sustained power output - clearly this is not necessarily the case. The point was also made that, as suggested by the early work of Goldspink, in shortening contractions at higher velocities fast muscle may be more efficient than slow muscle.

In relation to the talk by **Rome** the discussion included questions concerning:
- whether fish utilize elastic energy. It seemed that this probably would not be energetically important for the fast fibres because they are so seldom used and for very short periods.
- what the basis might be for inter-species differences in the relative amounts of "slow" and "fast" fibre types (histochemical types I and II). It was pointed out that for animals of the same structure and life style, greater proportions of weight-carrying "postural" fibres would be expected in a heavy than in a light animal because, in relation to linear body dimensions, force would increase by a power of 2 and weight by a power of 3. In accordance with such expectations, the percentage of type I fibres in antigravity muscles is higher for cats than for rats, and higher still for man than for the cat. However, the importance of other inter-species differences than variations in linear dimensions is underlined by the fact that no excessively high percentages of type I fibres are found in, for instance, limb muscles of the horse. Thus, in addition to variations in body weight, differences in body structure and in general motor behaviour are presumably also of great importance for muscle composition.

NEURONAL MECHANISMS AND PROCESSES

In relation to the talk by **Kernell** it was pointed out:
- that the afterhyperpolarization of motoneurones can be modified by synaptic means (e.g. effects of mono-amines) and that this represents an important mechanism for altering neuronal functions.
- that much is still unknown concerning motoneuronal plasticity; for instance, it is still unknown to what an extent fast motoneurones might change their properties as a result of a long-lasting increase in their amount of daily use

In relation to the talk by **Bigland-Ritchie**, questions were raised concerning the possible time-relation between the slowing of the muscle during exercise and the feeling of discomfort and pain; this problem is of interest because the afferents signalling pain may also be involved in reflexes causing a decline in motoneuronal (MN) firing rate. It was pointed out that, during exercise, slowed muscles hurt; conversely, however, muscles may hurt before becoming slowed. Similarly, metabolic changes take place at stages associated with muscle discomfort whereas, conversely, the sense of effort rises continuously also long before the occurrence of clear metabolic alterations.

Furthermore, it was pointed out that the time course of changes in MN discharge rate shows a resemblance to the concurrent changes in muscle fibre conduction velocity (CV), which are likely to be caused by metabolic influences. After ischaemic contractions and following the return of circulation, the fast recovery of MN firing rate and muscle CV would both presumably depend on the washing-out of extracellular accumulations of metabolites.

Later on (during the general discussion) a question was put concerning which metabolite might be leaking out of the muscle cells to cause the effects. It was suggested that the recovery of MN discharge rate after the release of ischemia was too fast to make lactate a likely candidate. Potassium ions were discussed as an alternative.

In relation to the talk by **Gandevia**, the discussion dealt with questions concerning:
- whether the last-recruited MNs of a voluntary contraction will normally ever reach the discharge rates needed for maximum tetanic force;
- the resolution of the twitch-interpolation method in cases of neuromuscular fatigue, which is likely to decrease the capacity for force-generation in fatigue-sensitive units. Hence, after a fatiguing exercise, the twitch-interpolation technique might lead to an over-estimate of the degree of MN activation during a voluntary contraction.
- the fact that very little is yet known about the MN firing rates during dynamic (shortening) contractions.

In relation to the talk by **Stuart**, it was pointed out by one discussant that, under dynamic working conditions, the slowed relaxation of a muscle may be functionally more important than the loss of maximum force (cf. alternating movements in swimming fish). In this context, the point was raised of whether it would not be easier for the central nervous system (CNS) to make use of some kind of mechanoreceptors for signalling fatigue-associated muscle changes rather than using afferents activated by metabolic products. Furthermore, general questions were asked concerning the extent to which segmental neuronal mechanisms might contribute to fatigue rather than helping to compensate for changes in the periphery.

GENERAL DISCUSSIONS

On several occassions there was discussion regarding the possibility of a central component to the fatigue seen in dynamic exercise. It was pointed out that there appeared to be differences between muscles in the ease with which maximal voluntary activation could be achieved and maintained, at least in isometric contractions. In a complex whole-body activity such as sprinting where many more muscles than those being tested may be involved it was suggested that there may be a role for central impairment. In response reference was made to a number of studies which have used percutaneous, or femoral nerve electrical stimulation, to confirm maximality of voluntary effort in shortening contractions. Given, however, the difficulty of these types of experiments one could not always *absolutely* exclude a central factor and prudence in interpreting results should be exercised. Nevertheless the accumulating evidence did suggest that it was not normally a factor. In relation to this it was also pointed out that during dynamic contractions the maximal force generated was much smaller than for example in isometric contractions (for example at 60 rev/min in isokinetic cycling this was less than 50% of maximal isometric force). This may be significant in relation to possible inhibitory effects associated with high force generation.Taken together this body of data seems to support the view that in dynamic contractions subjects are able, voluntarily, to fully activate their muscles.

-In relation to this issue it was pointed out that there was confusion and disagreement about how to deal with the question of central fatigue, but that it depended very largely on the question being asked. That is, are we asking if it is absolutely a mandatory component of all contractions? or, whether it is what people actually do do? When you look at a group of best efforts you almost always see some examples which show evidence of incomplete muscle activation, but equally, you generally have in each subject examples where they can fully activate the muscle.

There was also discussion concerning:

- the extent to which muscles normally engage in isometric contractions; it was pointed out that, at least in land animals, such long-lasting contractions are highly important for the maintenance of posture. Furthermore, (near-)isometric contractions are also important for joint stabilization in limb movements (e.g. slow walking).

- recommendations that definitions and measurements of fatigue should not only consider changes in force generation but also those of power output and alterations in the speed of relaxation as functionally important time-dependent changes in muscle function during and after use. Furthermore, when considering length changes of whole muscle (tendon-to-tendon) it should always be kept in mind that those do not need to correspond to the length-changes of the respective sarcomeres (e.g. muscle lengthening may be combined with isometric contraction of the sarcomeres).

- comments concerning the markedly multi-factorial character of neuromuscular fatigue, and that the precise manifestation of the fatigue is likely to be highly task-dependent. It remains a problem for much future research to define the precise relation between various tasks (e.g. differing in type and timing of contractile sequences) and the resulting time-dependent changes in neuromuscular (and related CNS) functions. In these investigations, it will be important to determine the "key sites" involved in the time-dependent changes associated with different motor tasks.

- comments that neuromuscular fatigue should be looked at as a normal component of movement and motor behaviour and not primarily as a "deficiency" of the system. The "down-regulation" of neuromuscular functions, as represented by what we call fatigue, often has a clear functional role in protecting sensitive links of the system from undesirable (and potentially dangerous) over-use.

- observations that there seems to be a rather gradual and diffuse borderline between certain muscle changes referred to as "damage" and some of those those called "fatigue". Some instances of so-called damage clearly concern changes of a reversible nature (e.g. some of the alterations in muscle membrane permeability) and may represent normal aspects of muscle behaviour during exercise.

- comments that it is not yet clear what the precise role is for (micro-)damage in the inducement of usage-dependent changes of muscle properties (muscle plasticity). However, it is clear that evident histological signs of tissue-damage are not a necessary precondition for muscle plasticity. Furthermore, it was pointed out that some aspects of muscle damage may become induced by primary damage to the capillary endothelium.

- recommendations that one should, in fatigue studies, be cautious when using results from electrically induced contractions to interpret fatigue of voluntary contractions; even at the same (submaximal) force level, muscle usage is likely to be markedly different in these two situations.

- the hypothetical phenomenon of "motor unit rotation" was extensively discussed. According to a suggestion made more than half a century ago, fatigue might be counteracted by letting motor units cyclically replace each other during a long-lasting contraction; now and then some "tired" units would fall out and other "rested" units would come in to take over. It was agreed upon by those present that, in spite of the popularity and viability of the rotation hypothesis, nobody has ever been able to produce any proof for its existence (many have looked, no clear evidence was found). Changes in unit selection during long-lasting contractions seem practically always to be associated with changes in the executed motor task (e.g. changes in the precise direction of intended force and movement). In weak contractions, single units may continue to discharge continuously during at least tens of minutes and, probably, for several hours.

- it was again emphasised that when combining experimental data from different species for the analysis of the relation between histochemical fibre type composition and function one should keep in mind that fibres of the same apparent type according to myofibrillar ATPase staining might still conceivably be markedly different in various contractile properties. It is, for instance, still uncertain to what an extent functional differences between type I and II fibres of man are analogous to the known functional differences between type I and II fibres of rats or cats.

Author Index